DR. PATRICIA A. MURRAY
Department of Periodontics
UMD-New Jersey Dental School
110 Bergen Street
Newark, NJ 07103-2425

ITI Dental Implants

Planning, Placement, Restoration, and Maintenance

Thomas G. Wilson, Jr, DDS

quintessence
books

Quintessence Publishing Co, Inc
Chicago, Berlin, London, Tokyo, Moscow, Prague, Sofia, and Warsaw

Library of Congress Cataloging-in-Publication Data

ITI dental implants : planning, placement, restoration, and
  maintenance / Thomas G. Wilson, Jr.
        p.   cm.
    Includes bibliographical references.
    ISBN 0-86715-260-5
    1.   Dental Implants.   I.   Wilson, Thomas G.
    [DNLM: 1.   Dental Implantation — methods.   2.   ITI System
WU 640 I89 1993]
RK667.I45I83   1993
617.6´92 — dc20
DNLM/DLC   93-5021
for Library of Congress   CIP

Editor: Patricia Bereck Weikersheimer
Production Manager: Timothy M. Robbins

Composition: Midwest Technical Publications, St Louis, MO
Printing and binding: Everbest Printing Co, Ltd, Hong Kong
Printed in Hong Kong

CONTENTS

Once again, with all my love, to:

My Mother

Penny

Trey

John

CONTRIBUTORS

All contributors are members of the North American Section of the
International Team for Implantology.

Hans Peter Weber, DMD, Dr Med Dent
Associate Professor of Periodontology
Director, Division of Implant Dentistry
Harvard School of Dental Medicine
Boston, Massachusetts

David Cochran, DDS, PhD
Professor and Chairman
Department of Periodontics
The University of Texas
   Health Science Center
San Antonio, Texas

Thomas D. Taylor, DDS, MSD
Professor and Department Head
Department of Prosthodontics
University of Connecticut
Hartford, Connecticut

Frank L. Higginbottom, DDS
Restorative dentistry
Private practice
Dallas, Texas

Hugh B. Douglas, DDS, MS
Associate Professor of Restorative Dentistry
Department of Prosthodontics
Medical College of Virginia
Richmond, Virginia

Leon A. Assael, DMD
Professor and Department Head
Department of Oral and
   Maxillofacial Surgery
Director, Oral and Maxillofacial
   Residency Program
University of Connecticut
School of Dental Medicine
Hartford, Connecticut

PREFACE

ITI (International Team for Implantology) is a multinational noncommercial group of clinicians, academicians, and researchers numbering approximately ninety who have come together to advance implant dentistry. ITI implants, which are grounded in more than nineteen years of research, provide a combination of surgical and prosthetic advantages not found in other implant systems. As the popularity of this system has grown, the need for a detailed, yet practical book on the clinical application of the ITI implant system has become clear.

This text is designed for the clinician who wants a concise, useful introduction to the ITI system. Information is provided on topics from fundamental to advanced. Subjects covered include: screening and evaluation of potential implant patients; guidelines for the proper choice of ITI implants; specifics on the surgical placement in both routine and advanced cases; guided tissue regeneration in combination with implant placement; prosthodontic approaches; implant maintenance; treatment of failing implants and complications; and case presentations to show your patients.

Given the nature of the work, it would be difficult to represent the opinions of all ITI members in a single book. Therefore, there may be some differences between our ideas and those of other ITI members. The ITI system is used throughout the world; because governmental policies differ and because they may change, the reader must verify these regulations. Although we have made every attempt to ensure that the information is current and accurate, it is the reader's responsibility to confirm particulars, such as drugs and their dosages, before utilizing the information contained in the book.

ACKNOWLEDGMENTS

I learned much of the information contained in this work from Dan Buser, Hans Peter Weber, and Franz Sutter, and I am in their debt.

Every book requires a great deal of input, advice, and constructive criticism. This work is no exception, and its content, context, and flow have been markedly improved by the contributors. Of special significance is Frank Higginbottom, who contributed many of the images found in the prosthetics chapter. Also of great assistance was the editing by Hans Peter Weber, David Cochran, Hugh Douglas, Tom Taylor, and Mike Newman. The International Team for Implantology and the Straumann Company provided assistance and kind permission to use graphic materials, and Terry Cockerham did an excellent job of constructing the remaining drawings.

And, once again, this project would not have been possible without Georgia Wright.

Thank you all.

1 ADVANTAGES OF THE ITI SYSTEM

The selection of an implant system may be based on many criteria. Advantages of the ITI system include the following:

- Only one surgical procedure is required.
- The restorative components for the system are strong and stable.
- The implant material is strong and bio compatible.
- The capacity of the bone to bind to the implant surface is superior to other available titanium surfaces.
- A number of sizes, shapes, and designs are available.
- Prospective and retrospective longitudinal studies confirm the efficacy of the ITI system and the titanium plasma-sprayed (TPS) surface.
- The simple design allows for fewer parts.

The use of a midcrestal incision retains all the original keratinized gingiva while the use of a trephine during placement of hollow implants reduces the amount of bone removed during surgery.

Surgical Procedure

One of the major advantages of the ITI system is that the implant is designed to be placed with its coronal portion emerging from the bone. This feature saves the patient from the trauma of a second-stage surgery, decreases the surgeon's chair time, and decreases expenses associated with additional visits.

Restorative Components

Prosthetic connections are crucial to the long-term success of an implant. ITI implants feature an abutment cylinder that binds tightly to the implant body and is very unlikely to loosen or fracture (Fig 1-1). This is preferred because if these two elements become separated (unscrewed) during function, bacteria collect and result in inflammation of the surrounding tissues (Fig 1-2–Fig 1-4). The elements are then susceptible to fracture, thus becoming nonfunctional. Studies indicate the tolerance for space between implant and abutment to be less than or equal to 10 μm for the ITI system.

Small occlusal gold screws used in other systems often break or loosen, causing maintenance problems for the restorative dentist. The larger diameter ITI occlusal screws and their unique design greatly reduce this problem, providing more stability and strength than other designs while still serving as stress breakers. In addition, prosthetic abutments with octagonal heads and prefabricated gold copings provide a multitude of prosthetic advantages with the ITI system.

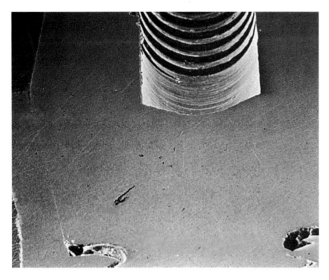

Fig 1-1   A scanning electron microscopic view shows the close interface between the ITI abutment cylinder and the implant.[15]

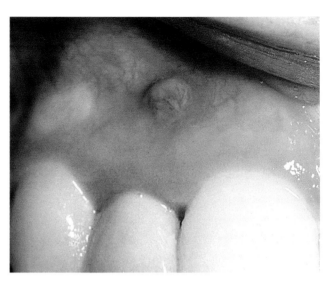

Fig 1-2   This patient presented with a fistulous tract around a two-stage (submerged) implant. The infection was caused by bacteria between the implant and the abutment cylinder. When the abutment cylinder was tightened, the fistula disappeared.

Non-rotation through mechanical lock

8

Morse Taper:
8° or less angle will yield a mechanically locking, friction fit.

Fig 1-3   The abutment cylinder and the implant meet at an 8-degree angle. This connection, called a Morse taper, greatly reduces or eliminates the possibility of a separation of implant and abutment, because it takes more force to remove the cylinder than to place it.

45° shoulder 30% smaller than 90° shoulder

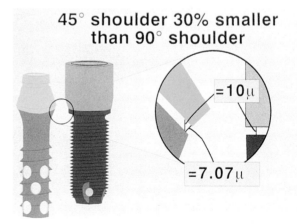

$=10\mu$

$=7.07\mu$

Fig 1-4   The 45-degree shoulder on the ITI implant reduces the microgap found between superstructure and implant when compared to a 90-degree shoulder. Note that with the ITI system the microgap is located just above or just below the soft tissue margin, not at the bone.

Implant Material

The material of the implant body and components should be strong. ITI implants are made from commercially pure grade-4 cold-worked titanium, which has proven most resistant to fracture.[1] In one test, 15-degree implants were subjected to 3,000,000 cycles of a 400 N/cm force, and no stress fractures or cracks occurred.

Tissue-Implant Binding

There are two widely used materials for implant-to-bone interface, titanium and hydroxyapatite. Hydroxyapatite has been shown to attach more rapidly and more completely to bone initially than does titanium.[2] This is due to bone growth from both the surface of the implant and the cut bone surface. With titanium, bone grows only from the cut bone surface. However, it seems likely that the degree of osseointegration to titanium increases over time,[3] reaching levels close to those found with hydroxyapatite.[4] Long-term problems with titanium may be fewer than with hydroxyapatite, since rapid dissolution of hydroxyapatite can occur when inflammatory cells come into contact with the coating.[5] A thin layer of hydroxyapatite designed to dissolve and lead to osseointegration on the underlying titanium may prove an alternative in the future, but at present titanium is the most stable surface coating.

The quantity and rate of bone adaptation to titanium depends to some degree on the implant surface's characteristics. Rough surfaces result in more rapid and more complete bone formation than do smooth coated implants.[4] At present, the ITI implant has a titanium plasma-sprayed (TPS) surface (Fig 1-5). This material is 30 μm thick with a porosity of 30–50 μm. It is chosen because it accelerates bone apposition,[6] increases bone-to-implant contact by up to six times compared to a

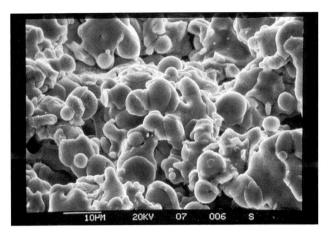

Fig 1-5 A scanning electron microscope view of the titanium plasma-sprayed (TPS) surface.

smooth surface,[4] and increases resistance to removal.[7] A sand-blasted, acid-attacked surface may prove to be superior to TPS if the results of initial tests on animals are borne out in tests on humans.[4]

The smooth titanium surface of the neck of ITI implants results in the formation of a tight collar of circular scar fiber of the subepithelial connective tissue surrounding the implant surface coronal to the bone, while the epithelium appears to attach in a manner similar to that found on a tooth.[8] Fears that these epithelial tissues would grow to or past the crest of the alveolar ridge during initial healing have been disproven.[8,9] It is of interest to note that in one study on dogs, the length of the epithelial downgrowth was significantly shorter in one-stage nonsubmerged implants than in two-stage submerged implants.[10]

Size, Shape, and Design

Shorter machined titanium surface implants (7 mm) have proven to be quite unstable in thin cancellous bone.[11] This is in contrast to ITI im-

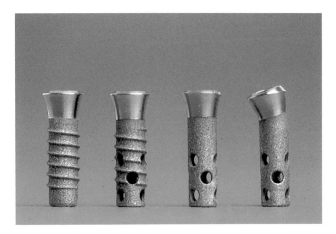

Fig 1-6   Shapes available for ITI implants, from left to right: the full-body screw (4.1 mm or 3.3 mm in diameter), hollow screw, hollow cylinder, and 15-degree hollow cylinder.

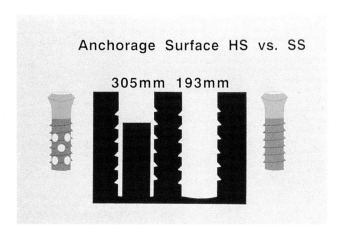

Fig 1-7   There is, on average, more than a 50% increase in bone-to-implant contact when a hollow implant (HS) is used when compared to a solid implant (SS).

plants, which have been successfully used in those situations requiring minimal length.[12]

Implant body shapes currently available for the ITI system include hollow cylinders (straight and with 15-degree angled heads) and hollow or full-body screws (Fig 1-6). The hollow implants have perforations 4 mm apical to the smooth collar. Implants with a screw design increase initial stability in thin cortical and cancellous bone and are recommended for use in these areas. Where the sinus or nasal floor is encountered, a full-body screw implant (available in 4.1 mm and 3.3 mm diameters) may provide some advantage.

Hollow implants provide significantly greater surface area for potential bony attachment than do solid designs (Fig 1-7), but have openings into the hollow inner core. These openings may prove to be an advantage or disadvantage. The advantage is increased bone ingrowth into the hollow section of the implant and increased resistance to torquing forces. The disadvantage is that if 4 mm of bone is lost around the implant (down to the level of the most coronal perforation), bacterial products may invade the inner portion of the hollow core, thus potentially compromising the future of the implant.

Efficacy

Prospective studies of the ITI implant system have shown high percentages of success, as have retrospective studies of the TPS surface.[12–14]

Other Advantages

The ITI system offers a number of economic advantages. First, when placed in the traditional manner, the system requires only one surgery. Second, the implants and equipment are moderately priced. Third, maintenance costs are reduced due to the strength of the system, resulting in fewer structural and prosthetic failures or complications. In addition, fewer instruments and components are needed for this system because several of these devices can be used for multiple purposes.

2 EXAMINATION OF POTENTIAL IMPLANT PATIENTS

Initial attempts at dental implant integration resulted in fibrous encapsulation of the implant due to overheating of the bone and instability of implant placement. Fibro-osseous implants (usually in the form of blades and subperiosteals) currently available have a failure rate of approximately 50% at ten years.[16,17] This failure is usually accompanied by a loss of a large amount of surrounding bone. While fibro-osseous systems may warrant reassessment as techniques for placement and materials improve, they presently have limited application and osseointegrated systems are preferred.

An understanding of the parameters involved in creating a wound in bone and the response of bone to the trauma allows osseointegration of dental implants to be routine. Osseointegrated dental implants are those that have intimate contact with the surrounding bone while in function.[18,19] This manifests as a "functional ankylosis" with no mobility of the implant when tested manually.[20] At present, osseointegrated fixtures are the implants of choice in the overwhelming majority of clinical cases because of their proven ability to function for many years[21,22] and because of their limited morbidity on failure. These devices have expanded the horizons of dentistry. They have allowed dentists to place firm dentures where none were previously possible and reduced the need for heroic measures to save teeth. While the clinician should make every reasonable attempt to save the natural dentition, osseointegrated implants often provide a more predictable solution to maintaining function than the use of severely compromised teeth.

Requisites for successful osseointegration include:

- Sufficient bone or the potential for bone to surround the implant
- Initial implant stability
- Adequate plaque control during initial healing (one-stage implants)
- Low-trauma surgery
- No functional loading of the implant initially

Communication Between Dental Professionals

The importance of communication between the restorative dentist and the surgeon is hard to overemphasize. The information gathered by each during the presurgical phase should be combined into a comprehensive treatment plan that allows for optimal results.

Screening Examination

Many patients are curious about implants. However, it is rare that the patient understands enough at the first dental visit to make an informed decision concerning treatment options involving implants. Because many of these patients are ultimately eliminated as implant candidates, valuable chair time will be lost if a detailed workup is performed on each new patient. Two strategies may help to avoid this problem. First, the patient can be provided with educational material (printed or audiovisual) before their initial visit as well as in the office before seeing the dentist. Additionally, the dental team can perform an abbreviated initial workup. This workup might include:

- A brief review of the patient's general physical health
  - Is the patient's cardiovascular system stable?
  - Does the patient have bleeding disorders?
  - Is the patient terminally ill?
  - Does the patient have an uncontrolled endocrine disorder (such as diabetes)?
- A screening oral examination
  - Does the patient have adequate oral hygiene?
  - Is there sufficient soft and hard tissue for implants?
- Radiographs of the implant sites
  - Periapical radiograph for individual sites
  - Panoramic radiograph for multiple sites

If the patient is deemed by the dentist to be a potential implant candidate, an overview of the implant process, an estimate of the fees involved, and alternative forms of therapy are then presented. If the patient expresses interest in continuing the process, a comprehensive examination is initiated.

Comprehensive Examination

Gathering information in the following areas should result in a set of treatment plans that include a full range of options from no treatment through the most comprehensive care. The advantages and disadvantages of each should be described, and ultimately informed consent on the part of the patient should be obtained.

Medical History

The patient usually completes a medical history which is followed by a dialogue on the subject between the dentist and the patient. Normal considerations for all dental patients should be evaluated as well as some additional factors.

Absolute contraindications to placing implants include:

- Uncontrolled endocrine disorder, such as diabetes
- Psychosis
- Abnormal wound healing that would result in implant failure
- Uncontrollable bleeding disorders
- Certain immune disorders, including HIV
- Other diseases or conditions outlined by the patient's physician, including certain cardiovascular disorders

Relative medical contraindications to implant placement include:

- History of head and neck radiation
- Cigarette smoking
- Other areas outlined by the patient's physician

When any doubt exists, the dentist should contact the patient's physician before therapy.

Dental History

The patient's view of his or her dental history is collected on the same written questionnaire as the medical history and is followed by a conversation on the topic with the patient. The patient's general knowledge, dental knowledge, motivation, and compliance must be considered.

The primary dental contraindications for placing single-stage dental implants include a lack of ability or willingness on the part of the patient to clean the implant, especially during the initial stages of healing after placement. This is important because one-stage implants are exposed to the oral environment from the time of placement. Lack of adequate bone and the inability to obtain more bone in the implant site(s) also contraindicates these implants. Problems could be caused by contiguous structures, such as:

- The nasal or sinus floors
- The inferior alveolar nerve
- The roots of contiguous teeth that cannot be moved orthodontically

  Relative dental contraindications include:

- Lichen planus at the site of implant placement
- History of head and neck radiation
- Uncontrolled periodontitis, especially aggressive forms (those seen in patients younger than 35 years)
- Retained roots
- Insufficient interarch distance

Comprehensive Clinical Examination

The extraoral clinical examination should include the following:

- Facial asymmetries
- Soft/hard tissue pathology
- Temporomandibular joint disorders

The intraoral examination should include examination of nonperiodontal soft tissues. The dental examination should include examination for:

- Dental caries
- Occlusal wear and patterns
- Restorations/prostheses
- Pulpal disease
- Tooth mobility
- Cracked or fractured teeth
- Occlusal habits
- Jaw relations (usually from diagnostic casts) (Fig 2-1):
  - Interarch distance
  - Jaw-to-jaw relationships
  - Tooth position and alignment

  Also examined should be the periodontal tissues.

- Periodontal or peri-implant tissues
  - Pocket probing depths (Fig 2-2)
    - Six per tooth
    - Up to six per implant
  - Gingival recession (Fig 2-3)
  - Disease activity
    - Increase in clinical attachment loss (pocket probing depth combined with gingival recession)
    - Bleeding upon probing/suppuration
- Amount of inflammation, plaque, and/or calculus
- Color, contour, and consistency of gingiva
- Furcation involvement
- Levels of adjacent cementoenamel junctions to implant site
- Amount of keratinized gingiva
- Frenum pulls
- Depth of vestibule
- Width and height of osseous tissue (may need bone sounding or appropriate radiographs)
- Thickness of gingiva

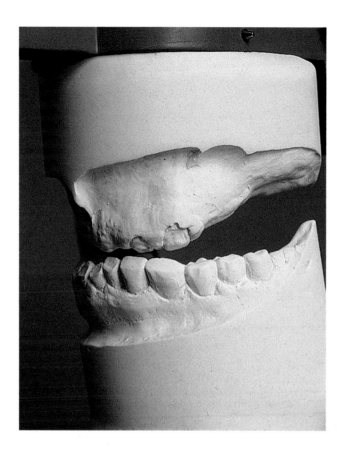

Fig 2-1   Study casts mounted on a semiadjustable articulator are helpful in treatment planning, especially to assess interarch distance and occlusal relationships. This patient had insufficient interarch distance, and bone was removed at surgery. (Study casts courtesy Dr R. Norman Dodson.)

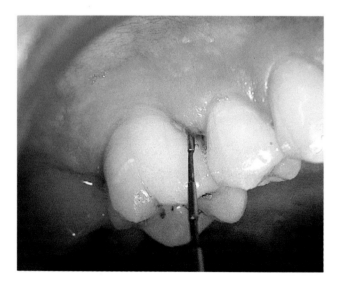

Fig 2-2   Six pocket probing depths should be recorded around each tooth, and up to six should be recorded per implant (a plastic probe is suggested for implants). The presence or absence of bleeding upon probing should also be noted and recorded, as should suppuration.

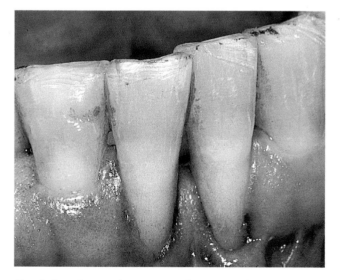

Fig 2-3   Gingival recession, if present, should be measured from the cementoenamel junction or apical margin of a restoration and recorded.

Template Fabrication

The long-term success of an osseointegrated implant is determined by the health of the surrounding tissues (peri-implantitis) and the prosthesis (access for oral hygiene and minimal trauma). The more optimal the placement and number of implants, the greater the likelihood of optimal prosthesis placement. Proper implant placement is greatly facilitated by preoperative construction and fitting of a surgical guide or template.

Templates can be of several varieties and be made from several sources, including:

- An existing prosthesis (Fig 2-4)
- A duplicate of an existing prosthesis (Fig 2-5)
- A vacuum-formed stent (Fig 2-6)
- A tooth-borne device similar to a habit appliance (Figs 2-7–2-9)

The use of templates is suggested in most cases. The more accuracy needed for implant placement, the more need for precise templates, which improve communication between the surgeon and restorative dentist.

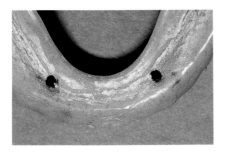

Fig 2-4

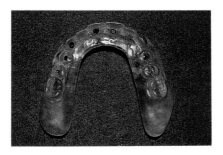

Fig 2-5

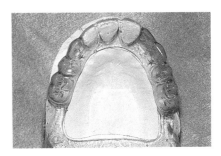

Fig 2-6

Fig 2-4   Access openings have been drilled in this patient's denture to serve as a surgical template. Openings are usually at least 3.5 mm in diameter to incorporate the largest bur or trephine.

Fig 2-5   This patient's maxillary full denture was duplicated in clear resin, and the palatal portion was removed to allow adequate space for the flaps. A connecting bar of acrylic resin is sometimes left at the posterior border to more accurately seat the template during surgery. (Template courtesy of Dr R. Norman Dodson.)

Fig 2-6   A template, vacuum-formed over a waxup or denture teeth placed in their proposed position, can be used during surgery. This type of template allows for more freedom of drill placement during surgery and can be used for areas where precise placement is not critical. (Template courtesy of Dr R. Norman Dodson.)

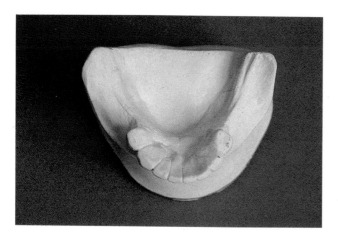

Fig 2-7   The patient's lower study cast before denture teeth are added to the proposed implant sites.

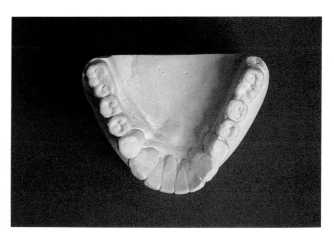

Fig 2-8   The study cast seen in Fig 2-7 after posterior denture teeth have been added.

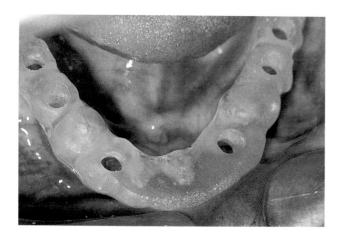

Fig 2-9   A template fabricated over the study cast seen in Fig 2-8. This template fits on the remaining teeth, and 3.5-mm access openings for guiding burs and trephines during surgery have been drilled.

Radiographic Examination

For patients with templates containing radiographic markers, one can use:

- Periapical radiographs (Figs 2-10 and 2-11)
- Panoramic radiographs (Figs 2-12 and 2-13)
- Lateral tomograms
- Computerized tomograms (Fig 2-14)

The clinician may occasionally feel that there is no need for templates. To view the bony housing in these cases, the following guidelines may prove helpful:

For cases that involve several implant sites, it is not unusual to use several different forms and angles of radiographs to have the maximum amount of information possible. Well-taken periapical radiographs provide the most accurate radiographic information and are suggested (possibly with other types of radiographs) in most cases involving partially edentulous patients.

Radiographic Examination Without Templates

Method	Indication
Mesiodistal/Coronoapical Dimension	
Periapical radiographs	• Single implants • Multiple sites where teeth exist
Panoramic radiographs	• As a screening device • A large amount of recipient site bone is anticipated • The floor of the nose, the maxillary sinus, or the inferior alveolar nerve needs to be located
Buccolingual/Coronoapical Dimension	
Lateral tomogram	• Single sites
Lateral cephalometric radiograph (Fig 2-15)	• Shape of the anterior region of totally edentulous mandibles with adequate bone height must be assessed
Computerized tomogram (Figs 2-16—2-18)	The clinician needs detailed information on the following situations: • Totally edentulous maxillary arch • Multiple mandibular or maxillary sites with minimal coronoapical bone height • Several potential implant recipient sites are planned

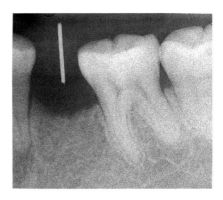

Fig 2-10

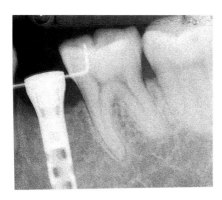

Fig 2-11

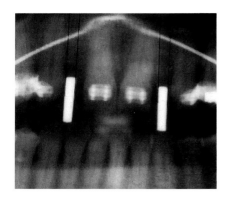

Fig 2-12

Fig 2-10 A radiographic marker (a piece of orthodontic wire) has been glued to a template. A periapical radiograph is taken, which indicates that the access opening should be drilled parallel to and mesial from the marker. (From an original idea by Dr Frank L. Higginbottom.)

Fig 2-11 The implant for the case depicted in Fig 2-10 immediately after placement.

Fig 2-12 A portion of a panoramic radiograph with radiopaque markers in place. The projection of these markers into the bony tissue predicts the insertion path of the implants. (Courtesy Dr Frank L. Higginbottom.)

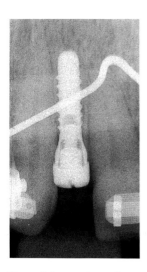

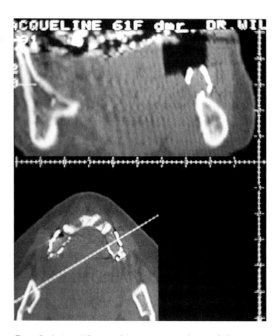

Fig 2-13 One of the implants from the case depicted in Fig 2-12 immediately after placement.

Fig 2-14 The radiopaque outline of the template shown in Fig 2-9. The outline seen in the upper right was made by painting the template with barium just before the computerized tomogram was taken.

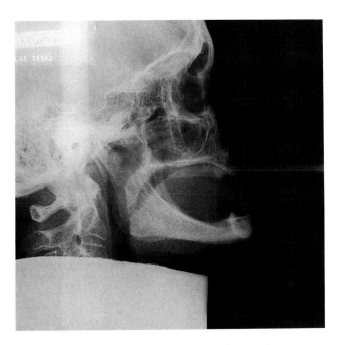

Fig 2-15 Lateral cephalometric radiographs can be used in totally edentulous mandibles with adequate bone height to help access anterior bone shape and quality.

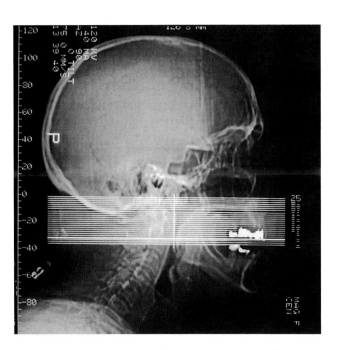

Fig 2-16 The dentist should request the scout film taken before a computerized tomogram to assure that the cuts taken were aligned parallel to the long axis of the jaw. If this alignment is off, the scan is not accurate.

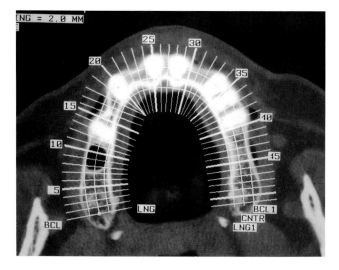

Fig 2-17 The numbered cuts seen after a computerized tomogram relate to the individual sections seen in Fig 2-18.

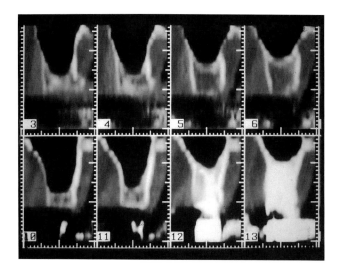

Fig 2-18 The program used after this computerized tomogram allows individual sections to be put in sequence and related to the overview seen in Fig 2-17.

3 TREATMENT PLANNING

Adjunctive Therapy

Once the clinical and radiographic examinations, histories, and consultations are complete, treatment planning can begin. While dental implants are an important part of therapy, it must be emphasized that they are only one part and one option. The clinician who makes treatment plans for dental implants only makes treatment plans in a vacuum. Many other aspects of dentistry affect dental implants and vice versa. Several of these areas of interaction are outlined below.

Periodontal Therapy

There is evidence that the microbiota found around a tooth with a healthy periodontium are similar to those found around an implant with healthy peri-implant tissues.[23] Teeth with periodontitis and implants with peri-implantitis also can have similar bacterial ecosystems. It appears that the tissues around osseointegrated implants in totally edentulous patients are healthier than tissues in patients with both teeth (with surrounding periodontitis) and dental implants.[24] This suggests some form of seeding of bacteria from natural teeth to implants. In addition, there is evidence that the danger of an aggressive form of periodontitis can be transferred to implants (Figs 3-1 and 3-2), this may be especially true in patients under 35 years of age.[25]

Additional evidence may prove or disprove these early findings, but at present one should proceed on the assumption that the microbes associated with periodontitis can be transferred to implants in the same mouth. This means that a thorough periodontal examination should be performed before implant therapy, and appropriate periodontal treatment should be rendered before or concurrent with implant placement. In cases of aggressive periodontitis, this will usually include traditional methods of therapy along with appropriate adjunctive care, often including antibiotic therapy and antimicrobial rinses. In patients with chronic forms of the disease, concomitant and continuing conventional periodontal therapy must be performed.

Endodontic Therapy

Endodontic therapy should be started before implant therapy in those areas where inflammation from the endodontic lesion could affect the implant site. In addition to reducing the probability of infection around the implant, this approach gives more information on endodontic prognosis before implant therapy begins, thus allowing formulation of a more comprehensive treatment plan (Fig 3-3).

Orthodontic Therapy

Orthodontic considerations are important in the treatment of implant patients for several reasons. *(1)* Placement of implants may alter orthodontic treatment. For example, orthodontics might be used to upright a second molar and then move it into a missing first molar site. With implant therapy, the tooth can be uprighted and an implant placed, saving the time and eliminating the stress of bodily movement of the second molar into the first molar site (Figs 3-4 and 3-5). *(2)* Osseointegrated implants can be used as anchorage for orthodontic movement.[26] *(3)* Once implants are integrated, they do not move. Therefore, any orthodontic therapy should be planned with the final implant site in mind. This often means delaying implant placement until after the completion of active orthodontic therapy.

Reconstructive Surgical Procedures

Reconstructive procedures must be planned with final dental implant placement in mind. The final implant placement and the success of the prosthesis depends on where the soft and hard tissues are placed at the time of reconstructive surgery (Figs 3-6—3-17).

Periodontal Therapy

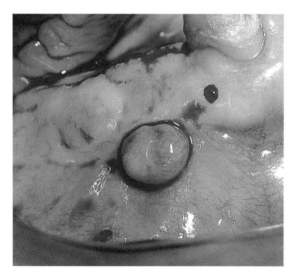

Fig 3-1

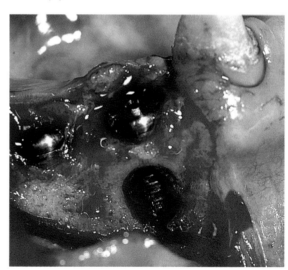

Fig 3-2

Fig 3-1   Implants were placed in a patient previously diagnosed as having refractory periodontitis. A few days after the implants were placed, the patient presented with localized swelling and tenderness around the most mesial implant. Various antibiotics were used, but the problem continued.

Fig 3-2   Thirty days after the implants were placed, the area seen in Fig 3-1 was opened and the mesial implant, which was mobile, was removed. Cultures were taken, an antibiotic appropriate for use during stage-two surgery was administered,[28] and the distal implant was successfully put into service.

Endodontic Therapy

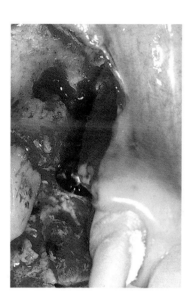

Fig 3-3   An endodontic lesion on the second premolar, undetectable on radiographs, was found to communicate with the implant site. The apical lesion was debrided, the patient was placed on penicillin, and endodontic therapy was rendered. Both the implant and the endodontic therapy were successful.

Orthodontic Therapy

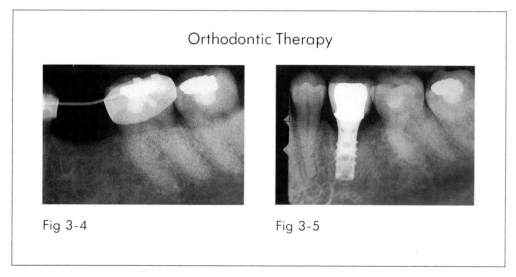

Fig 3-4

Fig 3-5

Fig 3-4   This tipped second molar was uprighted to avoid the necessity of torquing the root mesially. (Orthodontics by Dr Terry B. Adams.)

Fig 3-5   A single implant was placed in the edentulous space seen in Fig 3-4.

Reconstructive Surgical Procedures

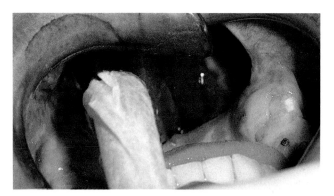

Fig 3-6   A young woman (at surgery with an endotracheal tube in place) had lost most of her maxillary teeth and hard palate to cancer surgery. In the ten years after the surgery, the periodontal condition of the remaining teeth had degenerated, threatening the removable partial denture and obturator that allowed the patient to chew and speak normally. (Figures 3-7—3-17 continue this case description.)

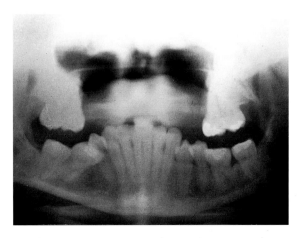

Fig 3-7   Preoperative radiograph.

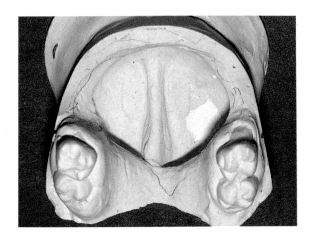

Fig 3-8   Preoperative study cast.

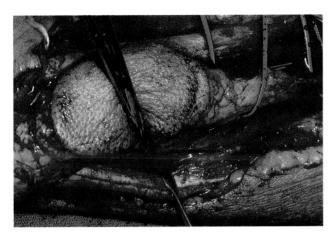

Fig 3-9 A composite graft of epithelium, connective tissues, bone, and blood vessels was removed from the patient's forearm.

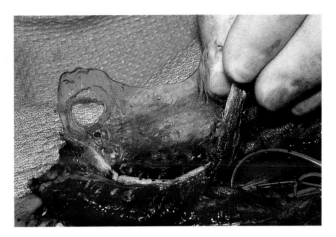

Fig 3-10 A template constructed on a preoperative waxup of a proposed prosthesis allowed the graft to be properly positioned. (Surgery by Dr Steve H. Byrd and Dr P. Craig Hobar; template courtesy Dr Frank L. Higginbottom.)

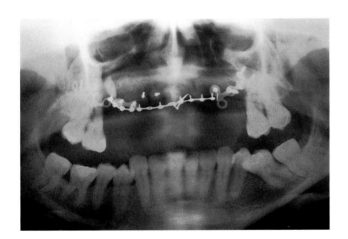

Fig 3-11 Radiograph taken just after surgery.

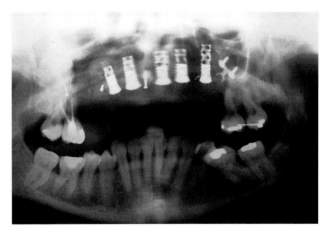

Fig 3-12 Radiograph taken soon after the first surgery. Five implants were placed; two failed due to trauma.

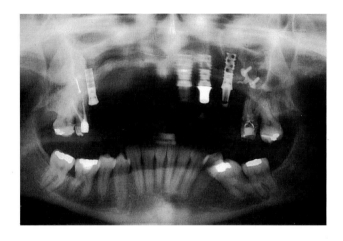

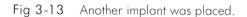

Fig 3-13   Another implant was placed.

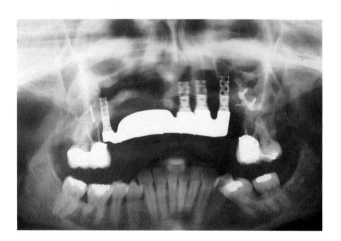

Fig 3-14   The laboratory model shows the final implant position.

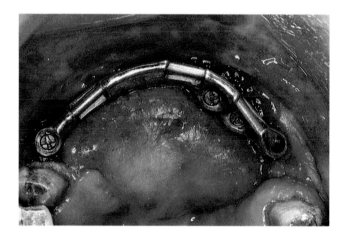

Fig 3-15   The bar is placed on the implant.

Fig 3-16   Final radiograph.

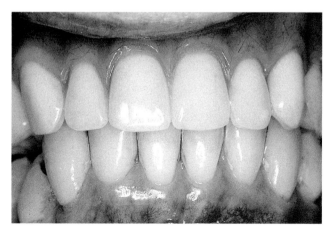

Fig 3-17   The final prosthesis, a bar-and-clip denture. (Restorative dentistry by Dr Frank L. Higginbottom.)

Selection of Individual Implants

The ITI system includes hollow cylinder, hollow screw, and full-body screw implants. Lengths currently available are 8 mm, 10 mm, 12 mm, 14 mm, and 16 mm, with 6 mm being used in Europe and the Far East and 4 mm prototypes being tested. The longest implant available that will fit into existing bone is normally selected. Implants of 14 mm or 16 mm are normally reserved for areas that will receive greater-than-normal occlusal forces.

Bone quality and width influence the choice of implant diameter. The diameter chosen should allow at least 1 mm of bone to surround the implant on all sides. Currently available diameters are 3.3 mm (full-body screw), 3.5 mm (hollow cylinder and 15-degree hollow cylinder), and 4.1 mm (hollow screw and full-body screw).

All come with a 3-mm–high smooth titanium collar coronal to the bone-anchoring titanium plasma-sprayed surface (TPS). The smooth portion is designed to extend through the oral mucosa. It widens coronally to a diameter of 4.8 mm, allowing the creation of a favorable emergence profile for most restorations.

The selection of implant sizes and types is based on the following:

- Coronoapical and buccolingual dimension of bone available
- Contiguous structures such as sinuses, the nasal floor, and the inferior alveolar nerves
- Distance between teeth contiguous with the implant site
- Quality of bone (Fig 3-18)

Fig 3-18 In Type I bone, most of the osseous tissue is compact. Type II has a thick layer of compact bone. Type III bone has some compact bone that surrounds a core of dense trabecular bone, while Type IV bone has a thin compact layer and low-density trabecular bone. This classification allows communication on the quality of bone, which is important because there tends to be a higher failure rate in less-dense bone.[11] (Drawing after Lekholm U, Zarb GA. Patient selection and preparation. In Brånemark PI, Zarb GA, Albrektsson T. *Tissue Integrated Prosthesis.* Chicago: Quintessence; 1985, p 202.)

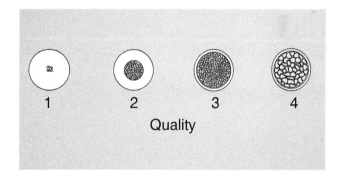

1   2   3   4

Quality

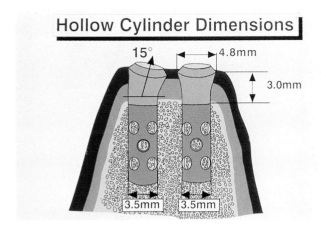

Fig 3-19   Fifteen-degree hollow cylinder (left) and regular hollow cylinder with dimensions.

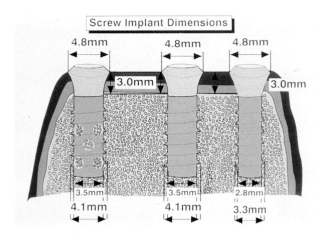

Fig 3-20   Hollow screw (left) and full-body screws with dimensions. Note that diameters of 3.3 mm and 4.1 mm are available for the full-body screw.

Indications for Individual Implant Designs

Hollow cylinders (Fig 3-19)

Regular hollow cylinders are usually used in sites where bone is dense enough to initially stabilize the implant (usually Type I or II bone).

Fifteen-degree hollow cylinders are used to redirect the screw channel of the octabutment or the long axis of the conical abutment. They can be used in any area of the mouth where initial stability and protection during the first stages of healing can be found.[27] This allows the implant to be placed in bone at a more ideal angle relative to the occlusal or incisal surface of the proposed prosthesis.

Hollow screws (Fig 3-20)

This design is normally used where additional initial stabilization of the implant is needed. This often occurs in Type III or IV bone, where the implant site has been enlarged during preparation, or when stability is not found with a smaller-diameter implant. This design also is preferred over the hollow cylinder in areas where bone density is minimal or in shorter implant lengths because of the additional implant surface provided by the screw threads.

Full-body screws (Fig 3-20)

This design is often used in sites 12 mm or greater where the additional retention of a screw is needed or when the solid body is thought by the surgeon to provide an advantage. These situations might include areas receiving guided tissue regeneration (GTR) or where the floor of the maxillary sinus or of the nose is penetrated by the apex of the implant. These implants come in 3.3 mm and 4.1 mm diameters.

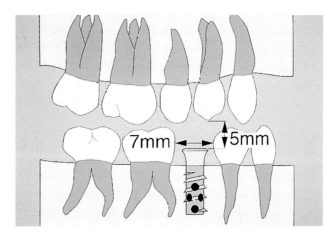

Fig 3-21 Dimensions needed for a single implant site.

Treatment Planning for Specific Situations

Single Tooth Replacement

Single tooth replacement can be one of the simplest or one of the most complex implant procedures (Fig 3-21). A single implant site should have:

- At least 1 mm of bone surrounding the implant on all sides, with 2 mm on the facial in areas of esthetic concern
- At least 5 mm interocclusal (interarch distance) measured from the top of the implant
- At least 1 mm clearance between the adjacent teeth and the widest portion of the implant (this means at least 7 mm between the teeth)

The site can be augmented to produce adequate bone if required.

A Tooth-retained Fixed Partial Denture vs a Single Implant

A fixed partial denture is chosen when:

- The patient prefers it to an implant
- The teeth on either side of the edentulous space are periodontally stable and need restoration

A single implant is placed when:

- A fixed partial denture would be unesthetic
- The patient prefers it to a fixed partial denture
- The contiguous teeth are not periodontally stable or the teeth have no restorations
- Large spaces or diastemas are present

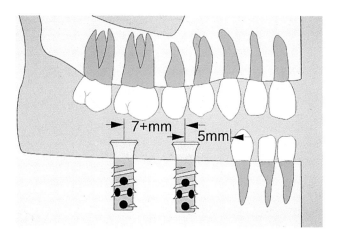

Fig 3-22   Dimensions needed for a partially edentulous site.

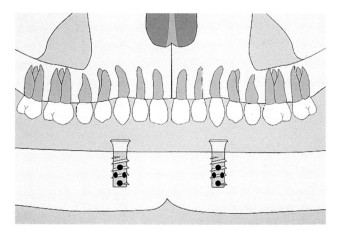

Fig 3-23   For implants with retentive anchors, the fixtures should be placed in the canine positions.

Multiple Tooth Replacement in Partially Edentulous Patients

To be successful, the implant recipient site should have (Fig 3-22):

- 1 mm of bone surrounding the implant on all sides, with 2 mm on the facial in areas of esthetic concern
- At least 5 mm interocclusal (interarch distance) measured from the top of the implant

Totally implant supported bridges are currently preferred over implant and natural tooth-supported bridges (ie, hybrid bridges). At least 7 mm should be allowed between implants as measured between their centers. Additionally, the center of the implant should be at least 5 mm from the adjacent root surface of any contiguous teeth.

Totally Edentulous Patients

There are three basic implant approaches for totally edentulous patients. Retentive anchors to support the prosthesis are recommended when (Fig 3-23):

- The patient is already wearing a denture and is comfortable with the concept of a removable prosthesis
- The patient wants or needs a device that prevents displacement of the denture, but allows the posterior areas of the denture to be supported by soft tissue
- Finances are of concern

Retentive anchors succeed best when:

- Implants are placed in the cuspid position
- The longest implants possible are used to achieve the greatest amount of support available
- There is an opposing denture
- Full-body screws are used.

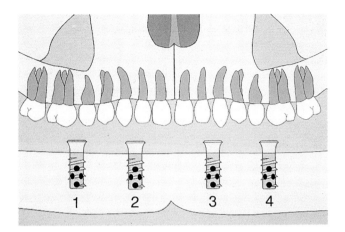

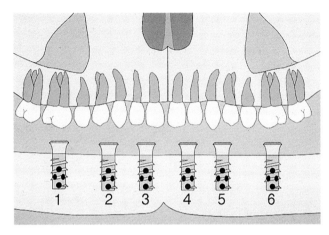

Fig 3-24   For a bar-and-clip—retained prosthesis, the 1 and 4 implants are best placed in the first molar/second premolar area unless the distance occlusal to the inferior alveolar nerve precludes an implant of at least 8 mm. Implants in the 2 and 3 positions are usually in the canine positions or slightly mesial to this position.

Fig 3-25   There are normally five longer (12 mm or longer) or six shorter (8 mm) implants used to support a fixed/detachable restoration. If five implants are to be used, the implant in either the 3 or 4 position is eliminated.

Use the bar-and-clip retained denture option when (Fig 3-24):

- The patient prefers a denture-like prosthesis
- The patient wants to eliminate the palate on a maxillary removable prosthesis
- The patient is accustomed to removing a denture
- The amount of bone lost affects the patient's speech or lip and cheek support and results in the need for a large base to support the prosthetic teeth, thereby compromising oral hygiene if a fixed/removable prosthesis is used
- The patient's present denture is causing soft-tissue damage and the patient or therapist wants to eliminate soft-tissue support of the prosthesis; four implants usually work well in these cases

Bar-and-clip retained dentures succeed best when:

- Two to four widely spaced implants are joined by a bar; at least 10 mm (on average) should be left between implant centers to allow room for clips to attach to the bar
- Clips inside the denture are placed in the anterior and posterior sections

Fixed/detachable prostheses are used when (Fig 3-25):

- The patient wants or needs the stability of a fixed prosthesis
- Available bone and soft tissue approximates, or can be augmented to approximate, the contours found when natural teeth were present in areas of esthetic concern

This option succeeds best when:

- The patient has good oral hygiene
- The implants are properly spaced and are of an adequate number

At least 7 mm should be allowed between implant centers. As a general rule, five longer (12 mm and up) or six shorter (8 mm) implants are needed per arch to properly support these devices. The longer the implants and the denser the bone, the fewer implants needed. The length of the arch and the force of the occlusion can also dictate implant numbers.

When the treatment planning phase is complete, a final consultation is held with the patient. Often several possible treatment plans, ranging from no treatment to comprehensive care, are covered with the patient at this visit. The advantages and disadvantages of each approach should be discussed, and the patient should be given enough information to make an informed decision. After the patient's decision, therapy begins.

4   IMPLANT SURGERY

Principles of Wound Healing

Bone

To aid bone healing, the implant surgery should allow for a close approximation of bone and implant. The bony adaptation to titanium results in osseointegration.[29,30] There are a few simple but important guidelines to follow to increase the chances for bony healing that will result in successful implants.

Overheating the bone kills or damages cells that will be important in healing.[31] To reduce this problem, the therapist should:

- Cool cutting instruments with chilled sterile saline either internally or externally
- Use slow drilling speeds (500–800 rpm)
- Use sharp instruments, which cut more precisely and with less heat than dull ones (on average, ITI predrills and trephines should be changed after the preparation of 12 implant sites[32])
- Use torque-reduction hand pieces
- Use an intermittent drilling technique when cutting with a trephine, (ie, periodically bring the instrument far enough coronally to rinse off and flush out any bone chips); if these fragments are not removed, the risk for overheating bone increases

To achieve optimal osseointegration, excessive functional loading in the healing period must be avoided.[33] Implants protected by contiguous teeth require only that the patient does not deliver any chewing or biting load to the implant for up to 2 weeks after placement and minimal loads for up to 3 months. Additionally, any overlying prosthesis should not touch the implant during the healing process.

Edentulous areas with implants that will be covered by full or partial dentures during healing should not be loaded for up to two weeks, if possible. If the patient cannot be without a denture for this time, the denture should be sufficiently hollowed out over the surgical area and be worn only as an esthetic device. After this initial healing period, the denture can be lined with a soft liner that is relieved around the implants. The soft liner is replaced when it hardens (usually after 30 days).

A stable implant, with close bone adaption at time of placement, aids in the healing process. In Class III and IV bone, screw-type implants can provide more initial stability than cylinders, especially in shorter sites. During surgery, the surgeon should keep the walls of the implant site as parallel as possible (ie, do not re-enter the bony preparation with the drill unless necessary). If the implant site has been widened during preparation, a screw implant is normally indicated because it provides greater initial stability.

Bone adapts well to the titanium oxide layer on the implant. This layer should first touch the patient's blood (usually in the implant site) when removed from the package. No other contaminants should be allowed to contact the implant surface because this may interfere with the wound healing process.[34]

Soft Tissue

The healing of soft tissue wounds can affect the ultimate success of the dental implant. A predictable series of events occurs following injury. A blood clot forms, and cells that clean the area of damaged tissues, foreign bodies, and bacteria are attracted to the wound. Epithelial cells begin to migrate from the wound margins and cover the fibrin clot. They continue to grow until they meet epithelial cells from the opposite side of the wound or come into contact with the implant surface. At the same time, fibroblasts migrate into the fibrin clot and a new extracellular matrix is formed. This fills in the wound and forms a scaffold for more cell growth and blood vessel formation. Over the ensuing days and months, maturation and remodeling occur until final wound healing is complete.

Instrument and Operatory Care

The rules for disinfecting the operatory and/or instruments are being constantly revised. It is strongly recommended that the surgeon and the rest of the dental team be aware of the latest methods and regulations for care of the dental facility as well as the dental instruments.

Implants are best delivered in a very clean environment, and the use of sterile barriers, drapes, and instruments is suggested.

Surgical Anatomy

Bone Resorption

In most cases, when teeth are extracted, rapid bone resorption and formation follows. While the amount and rapidity of bone loss varies from patient to patient, significant loss occurs in most patients (Fig 4-1 and Fig 4-2),[35-37] loss that continues over time.[38-40]

Maxilla

The incisive foramen is located just dorsal to nasopalatine papilla and contains nasopalatine vessels and nerves (Fig 4-3). The nerve supplies the lingual gingiva and the palatal mucosa from the canines forward. Nerve interference is usually not noticed by patients postoperatively, but cutting the vessels or their larger branches can result in bleeding problems during surgery.[41] Occasionally the foramen is so large that it precludes implant placement in the maxillary incisor areas. This can be especially true when significant periodontal bone resorption has occurred.

The greater palatine foramen is found medial and somewhat anterior to the maxillary third molars. The greater palatine nerve found here supplies the lingual gingiva and the palatal mucosa from the canines to the foramen[42] The greater palatine artery travels about halfway between the alveolar crest and the mid palate (Fig 4-3). Incisions (especially vertical ones) must be kept away from this vessel and nerve, especially in the molar areas, because the vessel can be rather large in some patients.

Lymph vessels for the vestibular gingiva drain to the submandibular nodes in both the maxillary and mandibular arch as does the palatal and lingual (mandibular) gingiva. This is clinically significant only when swelling, which may indi-

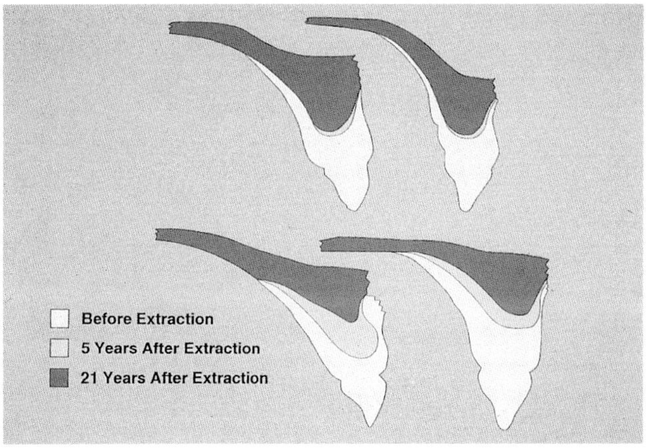

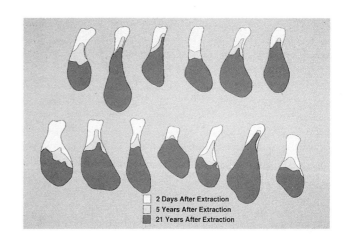

Fig 4-1 Bone resorption seen in these representative tracings of cross sections of maxillae on cephalometric radiographs in patients who received immediate dentures.

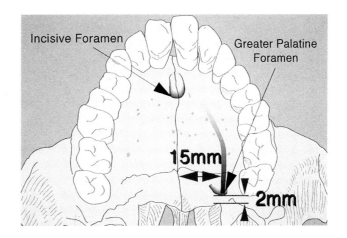

Fig 4-2 Tracings taken from cross sections of the anterior mandible two days, five years, and 21 years after extraction of the teeth in 13 patients. All the patients had maxillary dentures (Figs 4-1 and 4-2 drawn after Bergman B, Carlsson GE. Clinical long-term study of complete denture wearers. *J Prosthetic Dent* 1985; 53:56–61.)

Fig 4-3 The incisive foramen is located dorsal to and between the maxillary central incisors. The greater palatine artery exits the greater palatine foramen and travels anteriorly as its diameter decreases. Its course is usually midway between the alveolar crest and the mid palate (gray curved line).

cate infection, is seen in these areas post-operatively.

The floor of the nose and the maxillary sinuses can be often easily distinguished on radiographs. In practice, if these structures are penetrated, the implant is usually placed slightly inferior to or just at these structures, unless sinus lift procedures are performed simultaneously.

Mandible

One can occasionally feel the lingual nerve just lingual to the mandibular third molar. It arises from the floor of the mouth just medial to the root of this molar (Figs 4-4 and 4-5).[43] It supplies the dorsum of the tongue (anterior two-thirds). Vertical incisions distal and lingual to the second molars should be limited, if possible, to avoid this structure.

The inferior alveolar nerve[44,45] is an important structure to locate radiographically before surgery begins. A panographic radiograph is often helpful (Figs 4-6–4-8).

The mental nerve exits the mandible in the area of the premolars.[46] It is often helpful to locate this area during surgery of the mandibular posterior sextant to avoid damaging this nerve. By doing so, the clinician can more precisely measure the amount of bone coronal to the mental foramen (Fig 4-9).

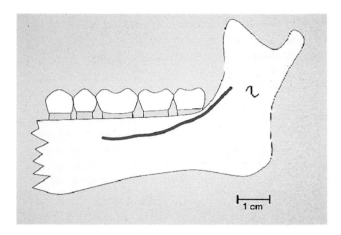

Fig 4-4   A lateral view of the average course of the lingual nerve.

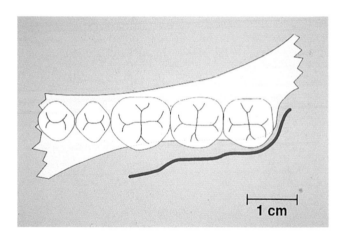

Fig 4-5   An occlusal view of the average course of the lingual nerve. (Figs 4-4 and 4-5 drawn after Wilson C. *Lingual Nerve: Anatomic Relationship to the Mandibular Alveolar Crest and Lingual Cortical Plate.* Thesis, Baylor College of Dentistry, Dallas, Texas, 1989.)

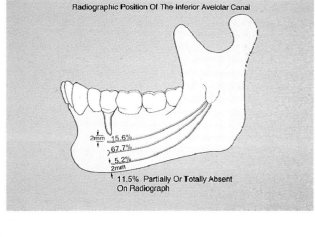

Fig 4-6   This lateral view of the inferior alveolar nerve shows the results of one study on its course: 15.6% of the time, the nerve was found within 2 mm of the apexes of the teeth; 5.2% of the time it was within 2 mm of the inferior cortical border; 67.7% of the time it was between these two extremes; and 11.5% of the time it was too indistinct to locate. (Adapted from Heasman PA. Variation in the position of the inferior dental canal and its significance to restorative dentistry. *J Dent* 1988;16:36–39.)

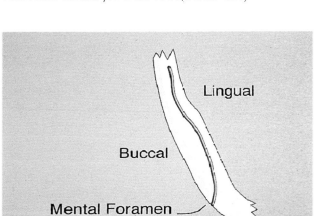

Fig 4-7   An occlusal view of the course of the inferior alveolar nerve.

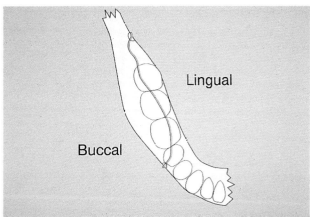

Fig 4-8   The same view as Fig 4-7 with the teeth superimposed. (Rajchol J, Ellis E, and Fanseca RJ. The anatomical location of the mandibular canal: Its relationship to the sagittal ramus osteotomy. *Int J Adult Orthod Orthognath Surg* 1986;1:37–47.)

Fig 4-9   Approximately 50% of the time, the mental foramen is located directly apical to the mandibular second premolar. It is frequently found 15 mm apical to the cementoenamel junction of this tooth. (Adapted from Matheson BR. *Localization of the Mental Foramen Utilizing an Intraoral Landmark.* Thesis, Baylor College of Dentistry, Dallas, Texas, 1985.)

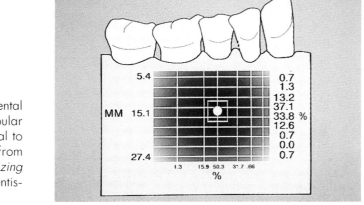

Instruments

The instruments recommended in addition to the ITI materials include a motor and hand pieces. The motor and hand pieces should provide low speed (below 800 rpm) and high torque. A motor with a pump for spraying normal saline on the drill is helpful but not essential. It is helpful because it reduces the need for a second assistant who is directly involved in the surgical field. The use of internal or external irrigation is the clinician's choice, since overheating of bone can safely be avoided by either technique when the procedures are performed according to the recommendations given earlier.[32] Hand-piece cords that can be autoclaved also are useful. Also recommended are a titanium periosteal elevator and a titanium curette. These may be helpful during implant placement, because touching the implant surface with stainless steel may compromise osseointegration.[47]

Instrument Replacement

Cutting burs and trephines should be replaced when they become dull, which, for the ITI instruments, is after the preparation of 12 implant sites in bone of average density.[32] The ratchet used to place screw type implants is regularly checked for proper function and is replaced when worn. It is best to keep a backup.

Basic Surgical Procedures

Preoperative Instructions for the Patient

Some clinicians like to administer antibiotics and analgesics before surgery. Some recommend ibuprofen (for normal adults, 600 mg every 6 hours for a total of eight doses) 24 hours before surgery. For the anxious patient, a sedative taken at bedtime and 1 to 2 hours before the surgical procedure may be prescribed (usually benzodiazapene). If intravenous sedation will be used during surgery, the patient should have nothing by mouth for 6 hours before the procedure. The exception is a small amount of water to take any needed oral medication.

The patient's physician should be contacted if questions arise about medications the patient is using.

Before surgery begins, the patient should use a mouth rinse of chlorhexidine digluconate for 30 seconds to reduce bacterial contaminants.

Standard Surgical Approach

For obvious reasons, an implant system that requires only one surgery is preferred over a two-stage approach. The ITI system was originally designed for a single-surgery approach with a flared smooth transgingival collar to facilitate the one-surgery approach. The following material details the conventional approach for placing hollow cylinders, hollow screws, and full-body screws used for the single surgery approach.

Hollow cylinder (Fig 4-10)

1. The thickness of the mucosa over the implant site should be determined before or at the surgical visit.
2. A midcrestal incision is made (or the remaining keratinized gingiva is bisected) (Figs 4-11–4-15), and the full-thickness flap is reflected. Bony contours are evaluated, releasing incisions can be used, and the ridge may need flattening or augmenting.
3. Cortical bone is penetrated by a series of round burs beginning at the exact center of the desired implant site. Use of a template is suggested but optional (Fig 4-16).
4. The longest predrill possible (for alignment purposes) is used to enlarge the opening in the cortical bone to a diameter of 3.5 mm. The drill is carried apically to its shoulder (Figs 4-17 and 4-18).
5. A trephine (again, the longest possible to aid in alignment) of appropriate length is used to prepare the site close to the desired depth (Figs 4-19 and 4-20).
6. An intraoperative radiograph is taken with the depth gauge in place (an optional step) if there is concern over anatomic structure or alignment.
7. The remainder of the site is prepared with the trephine. Conventional trephines are marked with depth holes or lines of 8 mm, 10 mm, 12 mm, 14 mm, and 16 mm. The line on the trephine should be at or slightly apical of the alveolar crest.
8. The depth is now rechecked with the depth gauge. The depth gauge is color coded. The colors match the colors on the implant containers:

Blue	=	6 mm
Brown	=	8 mm
Green	=	10 mm
Black	=	12 mm
White (silver)	=	14 mm
Red	=	16 mm

9. The implant-insertion device is placed on the implant and secured (Figs 4-21 and 4-22). The implant is then carried to the mouth and pushed into place. The implant-insertion device is removed. The implant can then be tapped into position by putting the implant-insertion instrument over the top of the implant and gently tapping the fixture to place. The TPS surface should be just covered by bone (Fig 4-23).
10. A large closure screw (healing cap) is placed (Fig 4-24).
11. The soft tissues are sutured snugly around the implant neck with nonresorbable suture (Fig 4-24).
12. Postsurgical radiographs may be obtained (Figs 4-25 and 4-26).

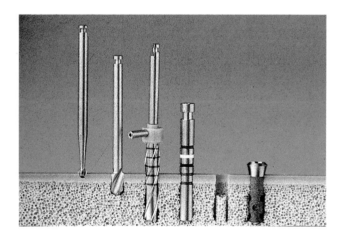

Fig 4-10 The sequence of burs used in placing the hollow cylinder implant. After the cortical plate has been penetrated by a series of round burs, the predrill and then the trephine (the internally irrigated model is shown) are used to prepare the site. The depth gauge precedes implant placement.

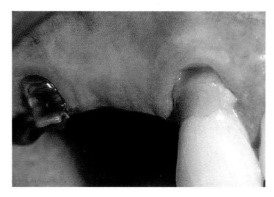

Fig 4-11   This patient lost a number of teeth from chronic adult periodontitis and dental caries. A single hollow cylinder implant will be placed in the position of the maxillary first premolar to serve as an interim abutment for a fixed partial denture.

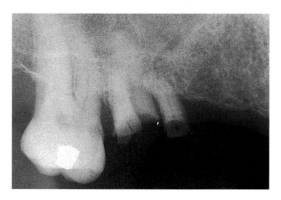

Fig 4-12   A preoperative radiograph of the proposed implant site.

Figs 4-13 to 4-15   Flap management for areas receiving implants.

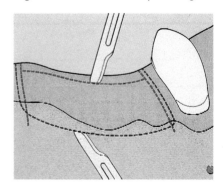

Fig 4-13

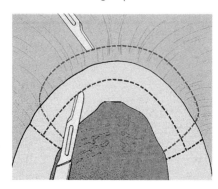

Fig 4-14

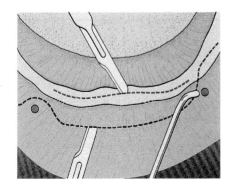

Fig 4-15

Fig 4-13   In posterior areas, midcrestal incisions are used for one-stage implant placement. Vertical incisions allow greater flap retraction, but they should be avoided if possible in lingual to lower second molar areas and palatal to maxillary molar areas. Use of the implant as a two-stage implant can involve the use of midcrestal (blue) or vestibular (red) incisions.

Fig 4-14   In totally edentulous maxillas, a midcrestal incision (red) with or without vertical releasing incision can be used for one-stage placement, while a vestibular (blue) or midcrestal approach can be used when the implant is used as a two-stage implant.

Fig 4-15   The totally edentulous mandible is approached in a manner similar to that of the maxilla except that the mental foramen is identified and avoided.

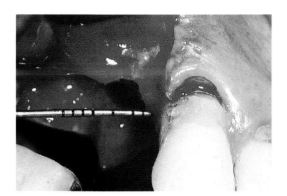

Fig 4-16   If a template is not used, the center of the implant is usually placed 5 mm distal to the contiguous tooth if bony anatomy allows.

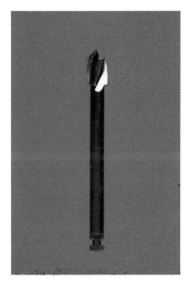

Fig 4-17

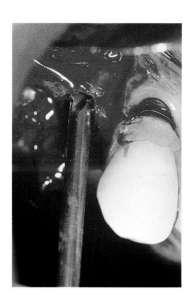

Fig 4-18

Fig 4-17   The predrill.

Fig 4-18   The predrill is started at the center of the proposed implant and carried apically until the shoulder is located just at or slightly apical to the bone crest.

Fig 4-19   The trephine drill. Two lengths are available, short and long. Use the long one whenever possible to allow for better alignment with contiguous structures. The trephine shown here has laser-etched lines. The instrument beside the trephine is used to remove any bone chips trapped during use.

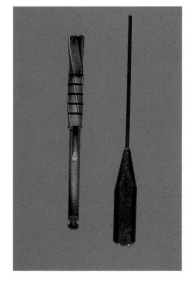

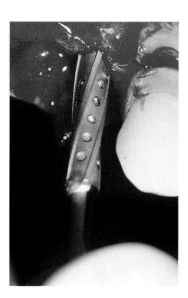

Fig 4-20   The trephine is marked in 2-mm increments, starting at 8 mm. The line that indicates the depth of the implant length desired should be taken just apical to the crest of the bone.

Fig 4-19

Fig 4-20

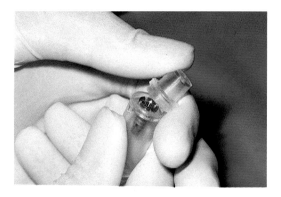

Fig 4-21   After being removed from its non-sterile outer package, the inner sterile package is popped open, exposing the coronal portion of the implant.

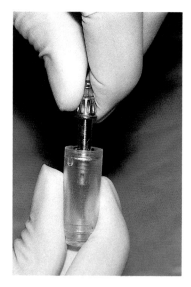

Fig 4-22   The implant-insertion device is screwed into the implant and tightened with the ratchet (arrow on ratchet facing the implant) and guide key. The implant is then lifted out and taken to the implant site. The implant-insertion device is removed, and the implant is tapped into place (if necessary) with the inserting instrument.

Fig 4-23   The implant is tapped into place. The TPS surface should be covered by bone.

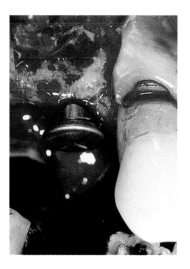

Fig 4-23

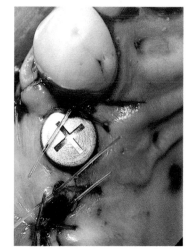

Fig 4-24

Fig 4-24   A large closure screw has been placed and the tissues gathered around the implant with chromic gut sutures.

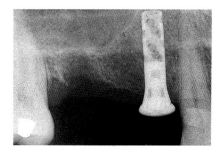

Fig 4-25   A radiograph taken just after implant placement.

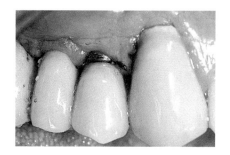

Fig 4-26   Two years after placement and immediately following scaling of the area. (Restorative dentistry by Dr R. Norman Dodson.)

15-Degree hollow cylinder

The steps are the same as for the regular hollow cylinder. This implant is used to bring the vertical axis of the abutment cylinder back into better alignment when the bony site is angled. This implant was originally conceived for use in the maxillary anterior region, but has proved useful in all areas of the mouth (Figs 4-27–4-29). The decision to use this implant can be made before surgery or during surgery.

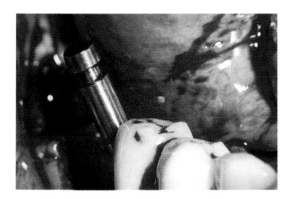

Fig 4-27

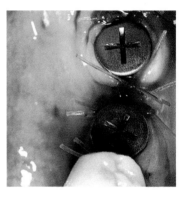

Fig 4-28

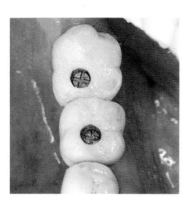

Fig 4-29

Fig 4-27   The first molar implant site in this case was angled to the lingual as demonstrated by the path of the depth gauge.

Fig 4-28   A hollow screw implant was placed in the second molar site and a 15-degree hollow cylinder in the first molar site.

Fig 4-29   The screw access opening in the occlusal surface of the first molar crown demonstrates that the vertical axis of the abutment cylinder was brought into proper alignment by use of the 15-degree hollow cylinder implant.

Hollow screw (Fig 4-30)

1. Steps 1—8 are the same as described for the hollow cylinder.
2. A tap is carried to the implant site and taken to the appropriate depth (Fig 4-31). The head of the tap should extend coronal to the adjacent teeth and stay above them when the tap is at the desired depth. Color coding on the tap indicates implant length.

   • In dense bone, the tap is taken to the depth of the implant preparation using the guide key and ratchet.
   • In less dense areas, the tap is taken just through the cortical bone.

   • Where little or no cortical bone is found, the implant is allowed to self tap.
3. The implant-insertion device is placed on the implant (Fig 4-32) and the implant is screwed in with the ratchet and guide key. The TPS surface should be covered by bone. In Class III or IV bone, the clinician may, as an alternative, want to place the implant by hand. The implant inserting device is used to turn the implant until it stops. Then the ratchet and guide key are used if necessary.
4. A large closure screw (healing cap) is placed.
5. The soft tissues are sutured snugly around the implant neck with nonresorbable suture.

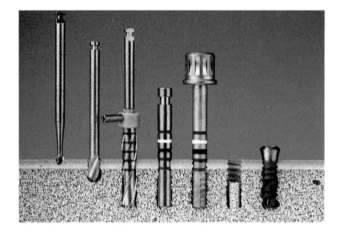

Fig 4-30   The initial sequence of burs used for the hollow screw is the same as for the hollow cylinder-round burs, predrill, trephine, and then the depth gauge. The tap is then used, followed by implant placement.

Fig 4-31   The tap is carried to the mouth in the ratchet and then taken to depth desired.

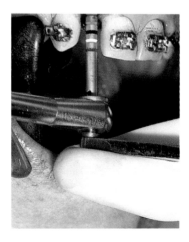

Fig 4-32   The screw implant is tightened with the ratchet (arrow toward implant) and guide key. The implant is then turned around in the ratchet and placed in the mouth.

Fig 4-31   Fig 4-32

Full-body screw (Fig 4-33)

1. Steps 1 and 2 are the same as described for the hollow cylinder.
2. The implant site is marked on the crest with round burs.
3. Pilot drill 1 (2.2 mm in diameter) is taken to the desired depth. Use of a template is suggested, but optional (Fig 4-34).
4. Pilot drill 2 (2.8 mm in diameter) is taken to the desired depth. Go to step 6 if a 3.3-mm full-body screw is to be used (Fig 4-35).
5. If a 4.1-mm full-body screw is to be used, take the 3.5-mm diameter twist drill to the desired depth (Fig 4-36).
6. Use the appropriate diameter tap for 4.1-mm implants and for 3.3-mm implants. Then follow steps 2–5 described for the hollow screw.

Using the techniques described for the hollow cylinder and screw implants, if the TPS surface is covered by bone and the soft tissues are less than 3-mm thick, the shoulder of the implant will rest coronal to the soft tissues.

In areas where esthetics is not a concern, if the conical abutment is to be used, the implant shoulder should be placed at or coronal to the soft tissue level. This placement facilitates impression taking and oral hygiene access later on, since the margin will be supragingival.

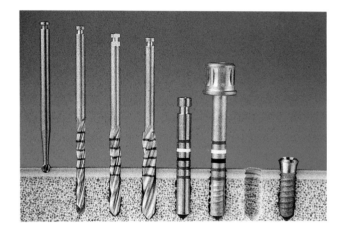

Fig 4-33   The sequence of burs used for placing the full-body screw is as follows: round burs, pilot drill 1 and 2 (for the 3.3-mm implant), pilot drill 1, 2, and 3 for the 4.1-mm implant, the depth gauge, and then the tap, followed by implant placement.

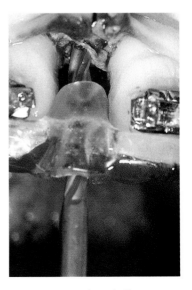

Fig 4-34   Pilot drill 1 in a stent.

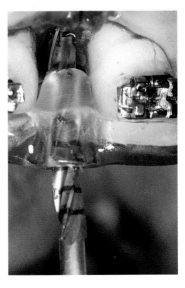

Fig 4-35   Pilot drill 2 in place.

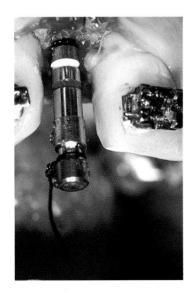

Fig 4-36   Depth gauge indicating a 12-mm implant.

Postoperative Instructions for the Patient

The patient is asked to adhere to the following postoperative guidelines:

- Keep the head above heart level for at least 24 hours
- Rest for up to 24 hours
- Avoid hot or spicy foods for 24 hours
- Avoid alcohol
- Keep an ice pack on the face for up to 24 hours, 10 minutes on, 10 minutes off
- Take antibiotics as prescribed (usually 10 days)
- Take ibuprofen and/or pain medication as prescribed
- Start twice daily rinses with chlorhexidine digluconate 24 hours after surgery

Immediate Postoperative Maintenance

At the first postoperative visit, usually scheduled 7 to 10 days after surgery:

- Check soft tissues for signs of infection
- Make sure patient is using chlorhexidine digluconate twice daily or is gently cleaning the implant with a soft bristle brush
- Remove sutures
- If healing is proceeding well, see patient in one week

At the second postoperative visit:

- Check soft tissues for signs of infection
- Advise patient to continue with chlorhexidine digluconate twice daily or gentle mechanical cleaning
- If tissues are healing well, see patient in two weeks

At the third postoperative visit:

- Check tissue for signs of infection
- Tell the patient, if the tissue is healing well, that they can stop using chlorhexidine digluconate
- Remove large closure screw and replace with small closure screw
- Advise patient to schedule visits at least every 30 to 45 days for three to four months

At subsequent postoperative visits, take periapical radiographs of the implants at end of healing period (three to four months). If implants are stable and appear without peri-implant radiolucencies on the radiograph, the patient is ready for the restorative phase. Implants placed in dense bone (predominantly cortical bone) are usually loaded three or more months after placement, while four or more months' waiting is used for those in less dense (more cancellous) bone. The patient should continue with postoperative visits every 30 days until restorative work is completed.

During all postoperative and maintenance visits, a rubber polishing cup with *fine* pumice or polishing paste should be used to remove plaque from the implant. This will prevent it from being scratched. If calculus deposits are found, they should be removed with special instruments to avoid scratching the implant surfaces.

Advanced Surgical Procedures

Multiple Implant Placement

Placement of multiple implants, either contiguous to one another or in other areas of the mouth at the same visit, offers special challenges. These procedures almost always require templates to properly position the implants. These templates are best constructed on models mounted on semiadjustable articulators. Proper positioning of the implants in relation to the proposed prosthesis can best be determined by placing denture teeth on the diagnostic casts. Proper planning and the use of templates during surgery optimize the end result. In many cases, one may want to parallel implants and not the adjacent teeth. Careful planning to avoid anatomic landmarks may be required.

Placement of the Implant in Esthetic Areas

Here the clinician must often modify traditional ITI placement techniques (Fig 4-37—Fig 4-48). If the ITI implant is used in the way it was originally designed, and the gingival tissues are less than 3-mm thick, the implant shoulder will be seen coronal to the margin of the gingiva. In many patients, this may be esthetically unacceptable, especially in the anterior sextants. To achieve a more esthetic restoration, a modified surgical approach is taken. The implant is apically positioned in the bone about 1.5–2 mm, and an extended healing cap is placed. One must remember to carry the shoulder of the predrill 2 mm apical to the most coronal margin of the bone. The trephine is also taken 2 mm deeper than the desired length of the implant. The TPS surface is therefore positioned apically by 1.5 to 2 mm. Transgingival titanium healing caps in heights of 2 mm to 5 mm may then be placed as an extension to the implants.

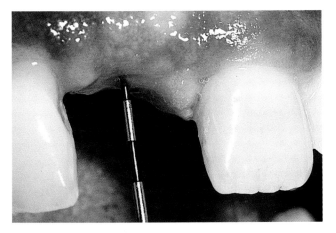

Fig 4-37 Presurgical probing shows the gingival tissue to be 3-mm thick. If traditional placement of the implant is used, the implant shoulder will be at the margin of the soft tissue. (This case is depicted through Fig 4-48.)

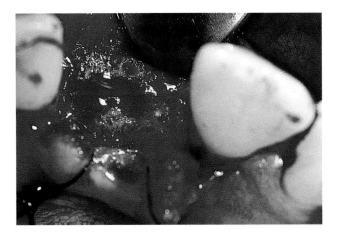

Fig 4-38 The initial opening with a small round bur was too far to the facial aspect, so the template was reworked and a second penetration made.

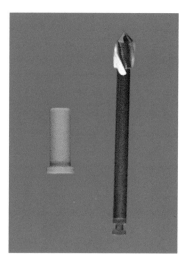

Fig 4-39   A predrill with a custom-made plastic sleeve to more accurately guide the placement of the drill was used.

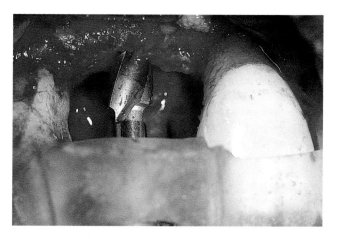

Fig 4-40   The plastic sleeve and predrill in the template.

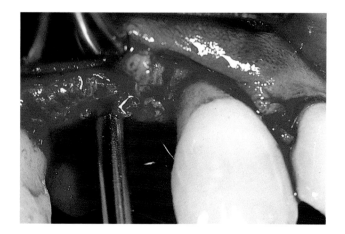

Fig 4-41   The predrill shoulder is carried 2 mm apical to the bone crest to allow more apical placement of the implant.

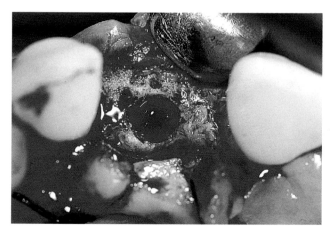

Fig 4-42   It is important to have approximately 2 mm of bone on the facial aspect of the implant in esthetic areas to reduce the chance for gingival recession.

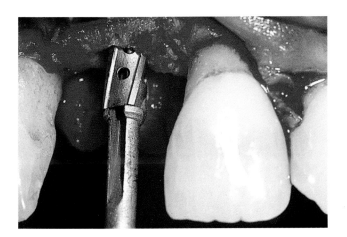

Fig 4-43   The trephine bur is taken to the 14-mm mark to place a 12-mm implant.

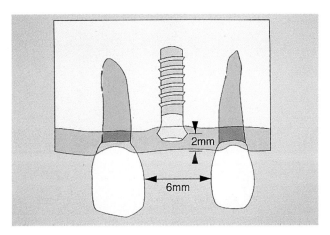

Fig 4-44   The implant is countersunk 2 mm more apically than in the traditional placement.

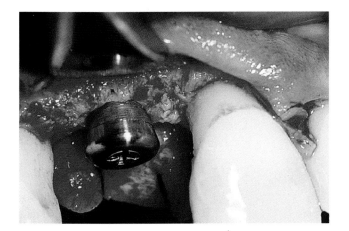

Fig 4-45   A 2-mm extended healing cap has been placed.

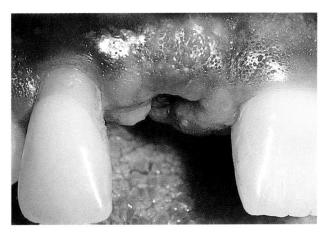

Fig 4-46   The soft tissues are sutured around the implant.

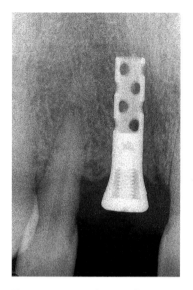

Fig 4-47   Radiograph taken immediately after surgery.

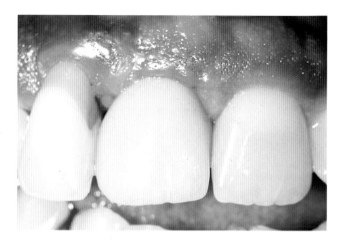

Fig 4-48   The final restoration. (Restorative dentistry by Dr Donald E. Dobbs.)

Placement of 6-mm Implants (Fig 4-49)

As this is written, 6-mm implants are available in Europe. They may later become generally available.

1. Determine the thickness of the mucosa over the implant site before or at the surgical visit.
2. Make a midcrestal incision (or bisect the remaining keratinized gingiva). Reflect the full-thickness flap, and evaluate bony contours. Releasing incisions can be used, and the ridge may need flattening or augmenting.
3. Instead of the usual predrill, use the 6-mm stop drill angle cut (Fig 4-50).
4. Follow this with the rounded-end 6-mm round cut stop drill (Fig. 4-51).
5. Use the 6-mm tap as other taps are used.
6. Complete the implant as described under basic surgical procedures, hollow screw, steps 2–5 (Figs 4-52–4-54).

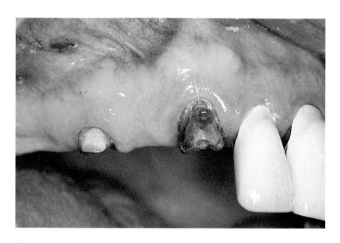

Fig 4-49   Minimal bone height in the maxillary first molar region and an opposing second molar occlusion dictated the use of a 6-mm implant.

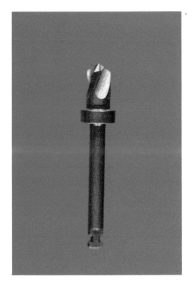

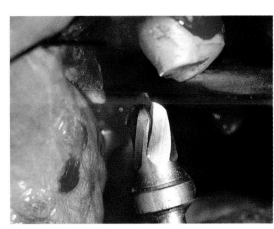

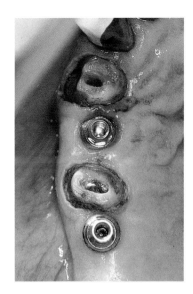

Fig 4-50   Fig 4-51   Fig 4-52

Fig 4-50   After the implant center is marked and the cortical plate is penetrated with a series of round burs, a 6-mm angle cut predrill is used.

Fig 4-51   This is followed by the round cut 6-mm predrill. Notice the flared ring on the drill, which limits depth penetration to 6 mm.

Fig 4-52   Four-months postoperatively.

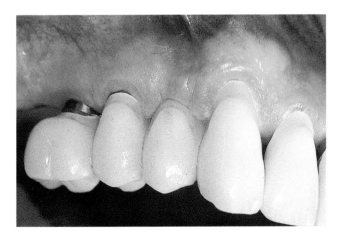

Fig 4-53   The final prosthesis. (Restorative dentistry by Dr Frank L. Higginbottom.)

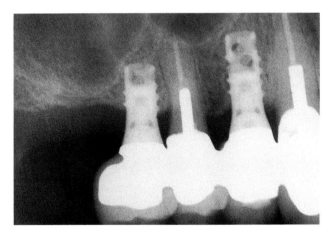

Fig 4-54   Radiograph taken approximately 2 years after implant placement.

5 GUIDED TISSUE REGENERATION

Guided tissue regeneration (GTR) is the use of a membrane to selectively exclude gingival tissues from a wound site, thus allowing the migration of bone or periodontal ligament progenitor cells into the area. In the case of dental implants, this technique selectively favors bone cells. This approach was first described for use around teeth.[48] Guided tissue regeneration is more predictable around implants than around teeth, probably because implants are sterile when first placed, appear to be impermeable to bacteria (titanium implants) and their toxins, only one tissue is involved, and the primary flap closure can usually be obtained. This approach, first proposed for use around implants in 1989,[49] has gained rapid acceptance. Most experience with GTR has been using e-PTFE (WL Gore) membranes, although other materials have been proposed.[50,51] While not all the questions about this approach have been answered, and infection has been a problem in some sites, the results are becoming quite predictable, and the procedure should be part of the implant surgeon's armamentarium.

The use of GTR can be broken down into four approaches based on its timing in relation to tooth extraction. These are termed immediate sites (Fig 5-1), recent sites (Fig 5-2), delayed sites (Figs 5-3 and 5-4), and mature sites (Figs 5-5 and 5-6).[52]

Immediate sites are those sites where an implant is placed at the same surgery in which the tooth to be replaced is extracted. Recent sites are those sites that have been allowed to cover with soft tissue after tooth extraction (usually 30 to 60 days). Because soft tissue coverage reduces the probability of membrane exposure and subsequent infection, the recent site is preferred over the immediate site. Delayed sites are those sites where GTR is used when the tooth is extracted and implant placement is delayed by some period of time. Mature sites are sites that need bone augmentation of a long-standing extraction site.

Immediate

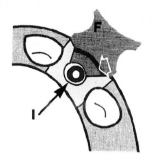

Recent

Delayed-Inital

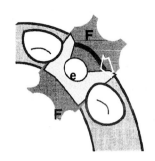

Fig 5-1

Fig 5-2

Fig 5-3

Delayed-Secondary

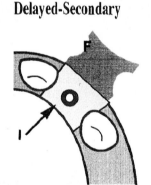

Mature Initial

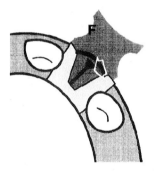

Mature-Secondary

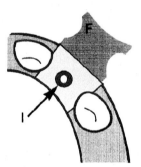

Fig 5-4

Fig 5-5

Fig 5-6

Fig 5-1   In the immediate site, the implant (I) is placed at the same surgery in which the tooth is extracted. A GTR membrane (arrow) is also placed.

Fig 5-2   In the recent site, the implant (I) and GTR membrane (arrow) are placed after soft tissue healing, usually 60 days following tooth extraction.

Fig 5-3   Delayed sites have a GTR membrane (arrow) placed at the time of extraction to prepare the site for an implant at some later date.

Fig 5-4   The implant (I) is placed after bone maturation in the delayed site.

Fig 5-5   The implant surgeon is unable to place a membrane at the time of extraction in the mature site, but in many cases the site needs ridge augmentation before implant placement.

Fig 5-6   The implant (I) is placed in the mature site after successful ridge augmentation.[52]

Recent and Delayed Sites

Tooth Extraction

1. Place the patient on antibiotics (starting 24 hours before surgery [optional]) (Fig 5-7).
2. Have the patient use chlorhexidine digluconate as a mouth rinse for 30 seconds just before surgery.
3. Gently elevate the soft tissues from around the tooth after the onset of local anesthesia.
4. Extract the tooth in the gentlest manner possible. Section multirooted teeth, if necessary. Avoid exaggerated buccal and lingual movements of the tooth to minimize trauma to the facial and lingual plates of bone, and avoid any removal of bone if possible.
5. Gently but thoroughly remove any granulation tissue from the socket.
6. Suture the soft tissues (Fig 5-8 and Fig 5-9). Obtain primary closure of soft tissues, if possible. In anterior esthetic areas, place sutures not in the papillary areas, but directly over the extraction site (Fig 5-10).
7. For recent sites, wait until the soft tissues mature over the extraction site before placing the implant. This is normally 30 to 60 days after tooth extraction (Fig 5-11). For delayed sites, GTR is performed at the time of extraction.

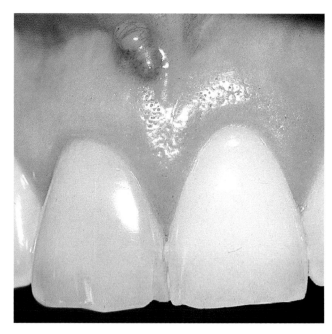

Fig 5-7   The right maxillary central incisor of this patient had failed to respond to treatment for external resorption.

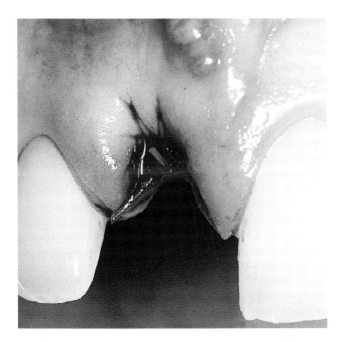

Fig 5-8   Since a recent site approach to implant placement was to be used, the socket was degranulated and the soft tissues were sutured gently together.

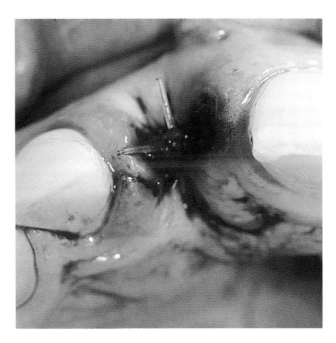

Fig 5-9   An occlusal view of the suture technique that avoids the papilla.

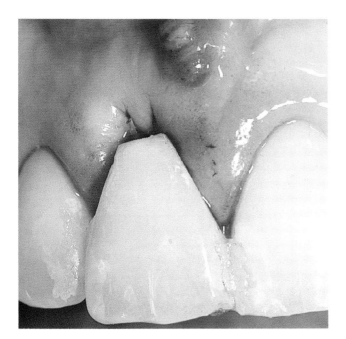

Fig 5-10   The coronal portion of the tooth bonded into position immediately after surgery.

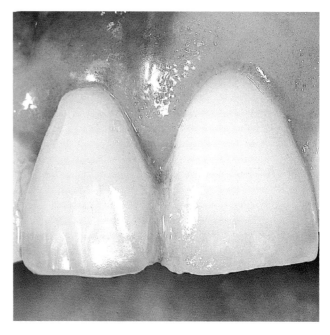

Fig 5-11   The area 60 days later ready for implant placement and GTR.

Implant Placement

In recent sites, the implant is placed 30 to 60 days after tooth extraction. In delayed sites, GTR is done at the time of tooth extraction. The implant is placed when the bone matures (usually 6 to 9 months later) (Figs 5-12–5-25).

If no GTR (or additional GTR in the case of delayed sites) is needed, place the implant in the most optimal position available and close the tissues in the normal fashion. If GTR is to be used, then:

1. Raise flaps that will keep the incision lines distant from the margins of the GTR membrane if possible.
2. Remove any soft tissues present in previous extraction sites.
3. Try in the membrane and trim it to cover the implant and bone defect and extend a few millimeters past the defect in all directions. Avoid touching teeth contiguous to the implant site, and avoid, if possible, the edges of the flap.
4. Put the membrane into place in one of the following ways (Figs 5-26 and 5-27): fix it to the implant with the cover screw; drape it over the implant; or drape it around the implant (cut a 4 mm hole with a slot on one side). This is the best approach.[53]
5. Ensure that the membrane rests in such a way as to create space between it and the bony defect and implant. This allows bone to grow underneath the membrane and can best be accomplished by:
   - The natural contours of the defect and the implant, or
   - Using small screws as "tent poles" underneath the membrane (Fig 5-18–5-27), or
   - Placing material underneath the membrane to hold space (such as autogenous bone) (Fig 5-14), or
   - A combination of these approaches[54]
6. Close the flaps and try to obtain primary closure. The flap should be tension-free to reduce the chances for tissue necrosis. It may be necessary to use periosteal releasing incisions and/or deep and wide reflection of the flaps. At this point in the procedure, the membrane *must* be covered.
7. If the overlying prosthesis is removable, leave it out for up to 2 weeks. If the overlying prosthesis is fixed, trim it so that no pressure is put on the healing tissue by the overlying fixed partial dentures used as provisionals. Care must be taken to allow extra room for swelling of soft tissues, which can be seen up to three days postoperatively.
8. The patient is told to adhere to the guidelines described in chapter 4 to reduce the probability of swelling, which is important because swelling may place tension on the flaps. The postoperative procedures are the same as those for non-GTR cases, except:
   - The membrane optimally stays in place for several months but it must stay in *at least* 30 days
   - If the membrane is exposed before 30 days, the patient is checked weekly and the membrane removed at 30 days
   - If the membrane is exposed after 30 days, it is removed when exposure is found
9. A total healing time of 3–6 months is average before the implants should be uncovered and loaded.

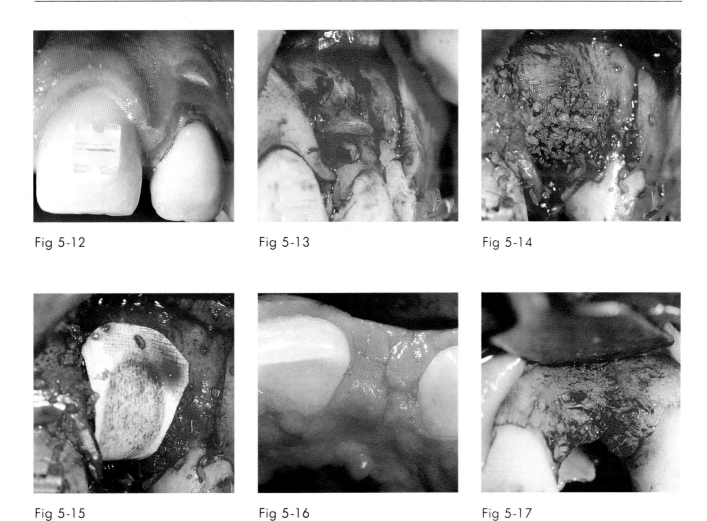

Fig 5-12

Fig 5-13

Fig 5-14

Fig 5-15

Fig 5-16

Fig 5-17

Fig 5-12   Endodontic failure necessitated removal of this maxillary lateral incisor. The delayed site approach was chosen because the patient was undergoing orthodontic therapy.

Fig 5-13   Moderate facial bone destruction was found when a flap was raised.

Fig 5-14   Freeze-dried bone to hold space was placed in the socket after tooth extraction and degranulation.

Fig 5-15   An e-PTFE membrane was placed over the socket extending past the margins of the defect for several millimeters in all directions.

Fig 5-16   The healed area at the conclusion of active orthodontic care. (Orthodontic care by Dr Terry B. Adams.)

Fig 5-17   The regenerated ridge can be seen just before implant placement.

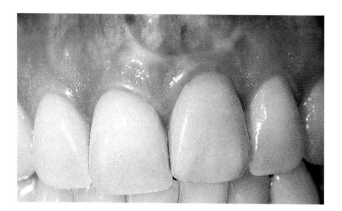

Fig 5-18

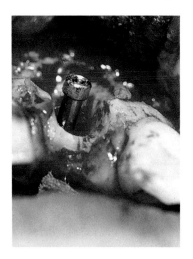

Fig 5-19

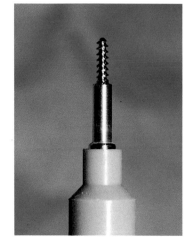

Fig 5-20

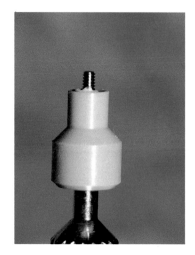

Fig 5-21

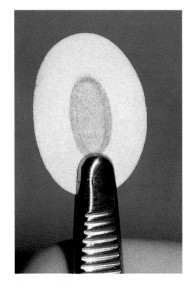

Fig 5-22

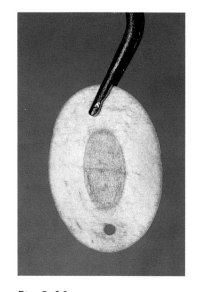

Fig 5-23

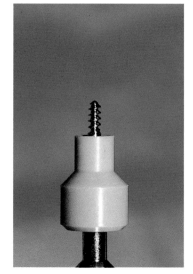

Fig 5-24

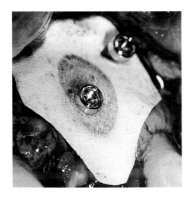

Fig 5-25

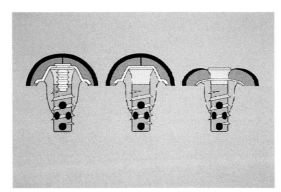

Fig 5-26

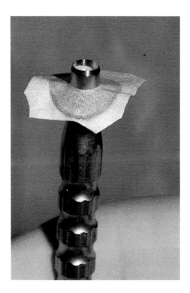

Fig 5-27

Fig 5-18   This patient's maxillary left central incisor was ankylosed and cracked. Extraction was suggested.

Fig 5-19   Insufficient bone remained for implant placement after tooth removal. A delayed site approach was adopted using a 3.5-mm supporting screw from the Memfix® System (Straumann Co.).

Fig 5-20   A 3.5-mm supporting screw from mini screw system in the screwdriver.

Fig 5-21   The head screw in the screwdriver.

Fig 5-22   Openings are made in the membrane with the 0.8-mm punch.

Fig 5-23   The opening made in a demonstration membrane.

Fig 5-24   A membrane fixation screw in the screwdriver.

Fig 5-25   The area after membrane placement. The e-PTFE membrane is fixed both to the supporting screw (center screw is the head screw, which attaches to the supporting screw through a hole in the membrane) and to the bone by a fixation screw in the upper right quadrant.

Fig 5-26   There are three ways to place the membrane over the head of the implant: left, attach it with an external healing screw; middle, place an internal healing screw and drape the membrane over the implant; right, cut a hole with the 3.5-mm or 4.1-mm punch and drape the membrane 1.5 mm apical to the implant shoulder.[53]

Fig 5-27   The membrane punch from the mini screw system is used when the surgeon wants to drape the membrane around the implant.

Mature Sites

In mature sites, the mature bone found at the proposed implant site is insufficient to house the implant. Therefore GTR is used to augment the ridge. Depending on the amount of available bone the implant is placed immediately or nine to 12 months later.

In mature sites, techniques for GTR described under recent and delayed sites are used, if necessary, to increase the amount of bone available for implant placement. In the mature site, these approaches usually involve the use of the mini screws mentioned earlier because of their unique ability to hold space under the membrane.[54] These mini screws are part of a system used to fix membranes during GTR. The kit (Straumann Co.) includes membrane fixation screws, screws to create space under the membrane, drills for creating locations in bone for screw placement and punches for making openings in membranes (Figs 5-28–5-34).

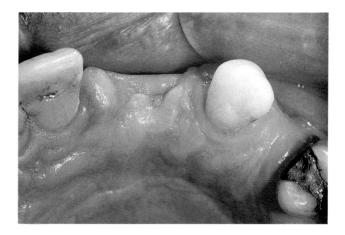

Fig 5-28   Teeth in this mature site were extracted several years before the patient presented for therapy.

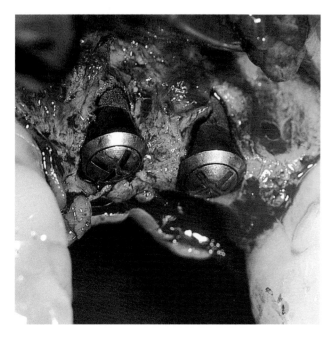

Fig 5-29   The facial aspect of the bony housing was less than 2 mm, and the TPS surface was exposed, necessitating GTR in this area of esthetic concern.

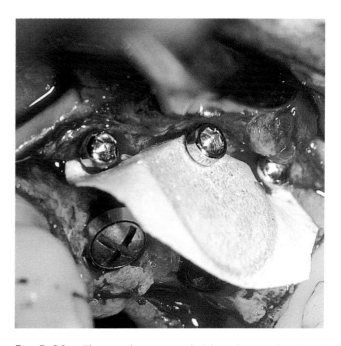

Fig 5-30   The membrane was held in place with a head screw attached to a 3.5-mm supporting screw (center) and two fixation screws (right and left).

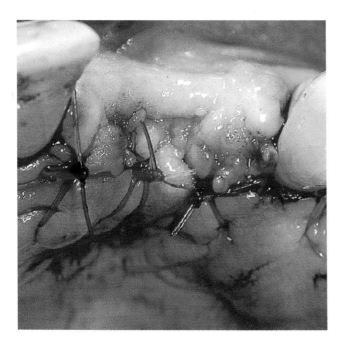

Fig 5-31   The area was closed primarily. Note the incision line at the lingual line angles of the teeth.

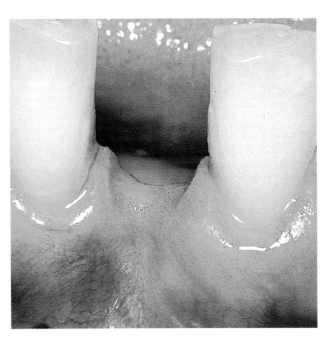

Fig 5-32   A mature site in the mandibular incisor region.

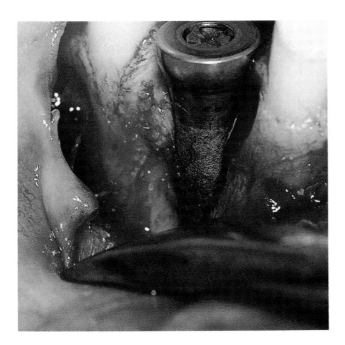

Fig 5-33   The implant at the time of placement.

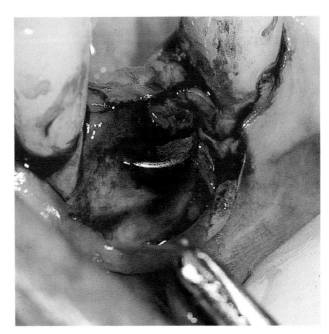

Fig 5-34   Clinical appearance approximately six months after placement. A flap was reflected and reveals a tissue that was solid when probed.

Immediate Sites

In immediate sites, the implant is placed during the same surgery in which the tooth is extracted.

1. The same techniques for tooth extraction described under recent and delayed sites are used (Figs 5-35–5-37).
2. The membrane is fixed in one of the manners described for recent and delayed sites.
3. Space is gained under the membrane in a manner similar to that described for delayed and recent sites.
4. Every attempt is made to gain primary coverage over the membrane.

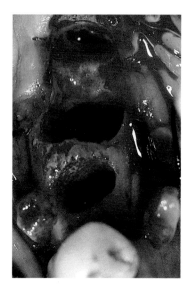

Fig 5-35 Immediate extraction sockets of a mandibular posterior area where the first molar and second premolar have been extracted and the sockets degranulated.

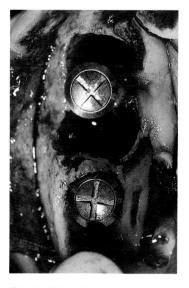

Fig 5-36 One implant is placed in the interfurcal bone of the molar and one in the extraction site of the premolar.

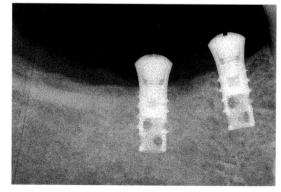

Fig 5-37 A nine-month postoperative radiograph. (Courtesy of Dr John ET Leonard.)

6 PROSTHETIC PROCEDURES

Restoration of the ITI implant usually begins three to four months after implant placement. Cases involving guided tissue regeneration (GTR) require a longer healing period (six to twelve months after implant placement before construction of the prosthesis begins).

Single crowns and fixed bridges constructed for ITI implants may be cemented or screw-retained. For cemented restorations, the conical abutment is selected.

Advantages of cemented restorations (conical abutment) are (Fig 6-1):

- Simplification of the fabrication of provisional acrylic resin restorations
- Reduction of the number of prosthetic components, therefore decreasing cost
- Decrease in maintenance because there are no occlusal screws
- Promotion of better esthetics because there is no screw access opening
- Intraoral modifications can be made before impression making

The conical abutment can be used when the long axis of the abutment lies within the confines of the proposed restoration. The conical abutment is available in two lengths, 3.5 mm and 4.5 mm. A minimum length of 3 mm is suggested after adjustments are made for occlusal clearance. Multiple splinted conical abutments can be used when implant divergence does not exceed 15 degrees.

The octabutment is selected for screw-retained restorations. A minimum clearance of 5 mm is recommended between the implant and opposing teeth.

Advantages of the screw-retained (octabutment) include the following (Fig 6-2):

- Restorations are more easily retrieved and modified.
- Splinted restorations may be fabricated with implant divergence up to 40 degrees.
- The impression for the master cast is simple and accurate because of precisely manufactured machined components.
- Restorations can be fabricated when the long axis of the abutment is not within the confines of the planned restoration (eg, custom-made angled abutments).
- Prefabricated gold copings allow a machined precise fit of the final restoration.

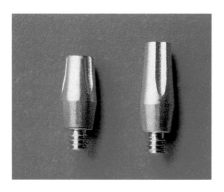

Fig 6-1   The conical abutment. Two lengths are available, 3.5 mm and 4.5 mm.

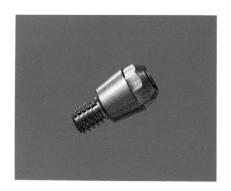

Fig 6-2   The octabutment.

Conical Abutment (Fig 6-3)

1. Remove the healing cap or closure screw.
2. Attach the conical abutment to the conical abutment driver. Using the ratchet and guidance key, tighten the conical abutment to the conical abutment driver (Fig 6-4). Insert the conical abutment into the implant and tighten the abutment hand tight. Using the ratchet, further tighten the conical abutment $1/12$ of a turn (30 degrees of a circle). This gives a tightening force of approximately 50 N/cm.
3. Using a copious air and water spray as a coolant from the high-speed hand piece, make whatever occlusal and axial adjustments are necessary for alignment and occlusal clearance.
4. Place retraction cord and make an impression with the impression material of your choice.
5. Make an opposing alginate impression; make a facebow transfer and appropriate interocclusal records.
6. Construct a well-fitting provisional acrylic resin restoration using vacuum-formed coping material constructed from a diagnostic wax-up (Fig 6-5). Cement the provisional restoration with temporary cement (Fig 6-6).
7. Box and pour the implant impression with die stone. Construct the restoration as you would for a natural tooth (Fig 6-7).
8. Remove the provisional restoration at the delivery appointment. Evaluate the restoration for fit, contour, proximal contacts, and occlusion. After appropriate adjustments, cement the restoration with the cement of choice.
9. Make a postoperative radiograph.

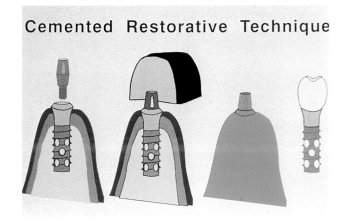

Cemented Restorative Technique

Fig 6-3 The sequence for a cemented restoration. Place the conventional abutment, take an impression, pour the model, and fabricate the restoration.

Fig 6-4 Tightening the conical abutment with $^1/_{12}$ turn of the ratchet stabilized with the key. The abutments have been reduced to allow for proper occlusal clearance.

Fig 6-5 The try-in for a vacuum-formed coping used in fabrication of temporary restorations.

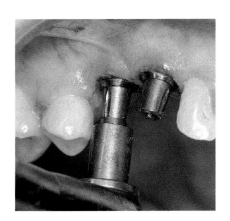

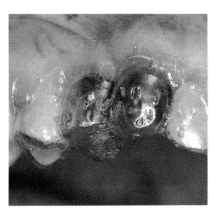

Fig 6-4

Fig 6-5

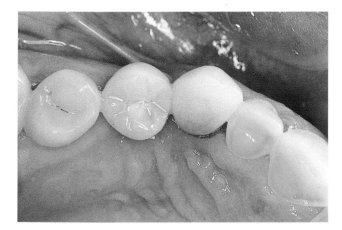

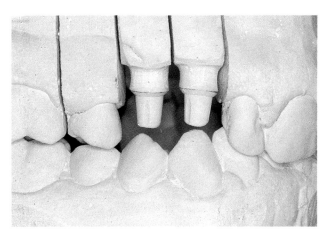

Fig 6-6 Provisional restorations completed.

Fig 6-7 Models trimmed and mounted on a semiadjustable articulator.

Octabutment (Fig 6-8)

1. Remove the healing cap or closure screw.
2. Place the octabutment in the octabutment driver and tighten the octabutment in the implant hand tight. Using the ratchet and octabutment driver, tighten the octabutment an additional $1/12$ of a turn (30 degrees of a circle). This places the octabutment with a force of approximately 50 N/cm.
3. Attach the transfer coping of your choice.

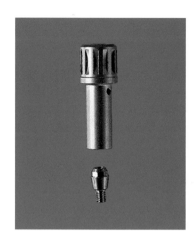

Fig 6-8 Octabutment and octabutment driver.

Construction of the Impression for the Master Cast

Two types of transfer copings are used in making an impression of an ITI implant. The repositionable transfer copings are removed from the impression, attached to an implant-abutment analog, and repositioned back into the impression. The serrated transfer copings are incorporated in the impression and are not removed from the impression when attaching implant-abutment analogs. Impressions using either type of transfer coping are quite accurate, and the type of transfer coping chosen is a matter of personal preference. A repositionable coping can be used for single crowns or when hydrocolloid is used as impression material. A serrated coping can be used for fixed partial dentures and bar reconstruction when impression material other than hydrocolloid is used.

Repositionable Transfer Coping (Figs 6-9 and 6-10)

1. Attach the repositionable transfer coping to the implant with an 8-mm raised-head occlusal screw using the occlusal screwdriver (Fig 6-11). Make sure the transfer coping engages the octabutment and fits flush with the implant shoulder.
2. With a custom impression tray, make an impression with an elastomeric impression material. Hydrocolloid may be used with this technique.
3. Remove the impression from the patient's mouth. Remove the 8-mm raised-head occlusal screws and the repositionable transfer coping from the patient's mouth.
4. Attach an implant-abutment analog to the repositionable transfer coping with an 8-mm flathead occlusal screw (Fig 6-12) and place the transfer coping back into the impression. The transfer coping should snap back into the impression, be stable, and have a positive seat (Fig 6-13).
5. Box and pour the impression with die stone.
6. Separate the impression and remove the flat head occlusal screw and repositionable transfer coping (see page 79).

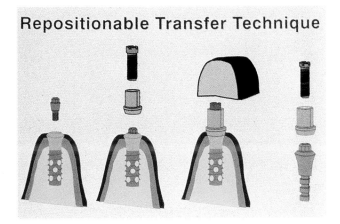

Repositionable Transfer Technique

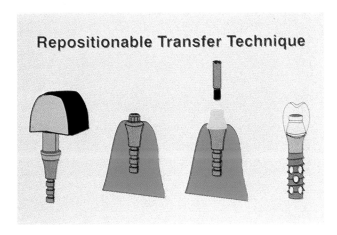

Repositionable Transfer Technique

Fig 6-9   The sequence for using the repositionable transfer coping (RTC) to fabricate a screw-retained prosthesis. Place the octabutment, retain the RTC to the implant with an 8-mm raised-head transfer coping screw, take an impression, unscrew the RTC from the mouth, and attach the laboratory analog to the RTC with a flathead 8-mm impression coping screw.

Fig 6-10   (Continued from Fig 6-9.) Place the joined RTC/lab analog into the impression, pour the model, fabricate the restoration, and place the restoration.

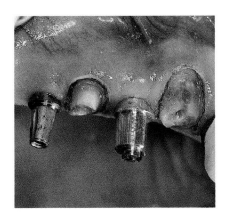

Fig 6-11

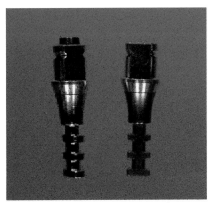

Fig 6-12

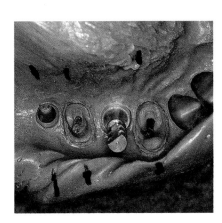

Fig 6-13

Fig 6-11   The repositionable transfer coping held in place by an 8-mm raised-head transfer coping screw.

Fig 6-12   The laboratory analog and the repositionable transfer coping attached with the 8-mm raised-head impression coping screw (left) and a flathead screw (right).

Fig 6-13   The joined repositionable transfer coping/analog unit placed into the impression.

Serrated Transfer Coping (Figs 6-14 and 6-15)

1. Attach the serrated transfer coping (also called the nonrepositionable transfer coping) to the octabutment with a guide screw using the occlusal screwdriver. Guide screws are available in lengths of 10 mm, 12 mm, 14 mm, and 16 mm (Figs 6-16–6-18). A guide screw length is chosen so that the screw penetrates through the impression tray. This allows the screw to be loosened after making the impression. Make sure the serrated transfer coping engages the octabutment and the transfer coping fits flush with the implant shoulder.
2. Try the custom impression tray in the patient's mouth and mark the area where the guide screws will penetrate the impression tray (Fig 6-19). Drill holes in the tray in these locations (Fig 6-20). Try the tray back in the patient's mouth to verify the size and location of guide screw holes in the tray.
3. Make an impression with an elastomeric impression material (Fig 6-21) other than hydrocolloid.
4. Unscrew the guide screws and remove the impression from the patient's mouth.
5. Attach an implant abutment analog to the serrated transfer coping with the same guide screw used for making the impression (Fig 6-22).
6. Box the impression with boxing wax and pour the impression with die stone.
7. After the stone has set, unscrew the guide screws and remove the impression from the master cast (see page 79).

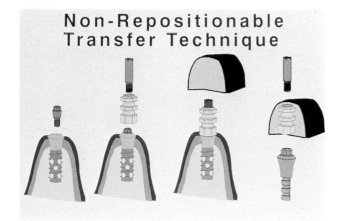

Fig 6-14 The nonrepositionable transfer technique. First, the octabutment is placed, then the serrated transfer coping, also called the nonrepositionable transfer coping (NRTC), is screwed in place with the guide screw. An impression is then taken, the guide screw is removed after the impression material is set, and a laboratory analog is attached to the NRTC in the impression with a guide screw.

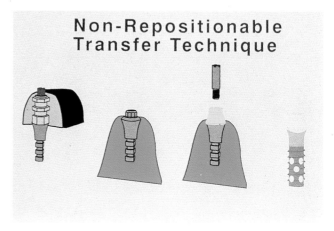

Fig 6-15 (Nonrepositionable transfer technique continued.) The stone model is poured, the final waxup is fabricated on a gold coping held in place by a guide screw, and the final restoration is fabricated and placed.

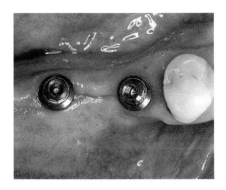

Fig 6-16

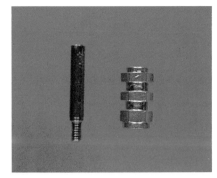

Fig 6-17

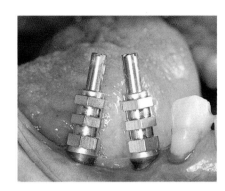

Fig 6-18

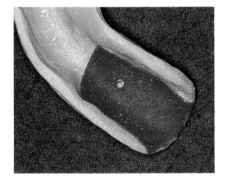

Fig 6-19

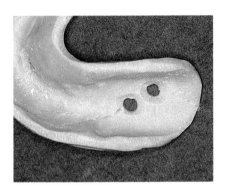

Fig 6-20

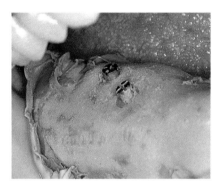

Fig 6-21

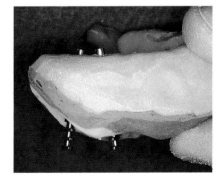

Fig 6-22

Fig 6-16   Octabutments in place.

Fig 6-17   The NRTC and a guide screw.

Fig 6-18   The nonrepositional transfer copings (NRTC) attached to the octabutment with a guide screw.

Fig 6-19   Marks made by the occlusal surface of a guide screw on boxing wax placed in the custom tray.

Fig 6-20   Holes in the impression tray made to correspond to the marks made by the guide screws.

Fig 6-21   Guide screws protruding through the custom tray when the impression has been properly positioned.

Fig 6-22   The guide screws have been removed and the impression taken from the mouth. The same guide screws are then used to hold an octabutment analog in proper relation to the NRTC. The NRTC is retained in the impression material.

Provisional Restorations Using the Octabutment

In cases where esthetics and function are not critical, temporary protective caps can be used to cover the octabutment. The smooth rounded contour of the temporary protective cap provides patient comfort and prevents food and debris from entering the screw access opening of the octabutment. A 4-mm occlusal screw is used to retain the temporary protective cap.

For cases where function or esthetics are more critical, a screw-retained provisional acrylic resin restoration can be fabricated.

1. Attach a temporary stainless steel coping to the octabutment with a 4-mm occlusal screw. Two types of temporary stainless steel copings are available: "octagonal" copings for single crowns and "rounded" copings for splinted restorations. Plastic temporization copings are also available (Fig 6-23).
2. Adjust the height of the temporary coping for occlusion. Intraoral adjustment should be made with copious irrigation to prevent overheating of the implant.

3. Place cotton soaked with petroleum jelly in the occlusal opening of the temporary coping.
4. Cut an occlusal opening in a vacuum-formed coping constructed from a duplicate model of the diagnostic wax-up (Fig 6-24).
5. Fill the vacuum-formed coping with autopolymerized provisional acrylic resin.
6. Remove the plastic coping and acrylic resin before the acrylic resin becomes hot. An air-and-water spray will help ensure that the acrylic resin does not get too warm. Reline and adjust the provisional acrylic resin restoration as needed.
7. Check and adjust occlusion, fit, and contour of the provisional restoration.
8. Polish the provisional restoration and place it with a 4-mm occlusal screw.
9. Place cotton over the head of the occlusal screw and close the occlusal screw access opening with temporary endodontic stopping, or acrylic resin (Fig 6-25).

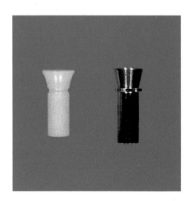

Fig 6-23 Metal (right) and plastic temporization copings.

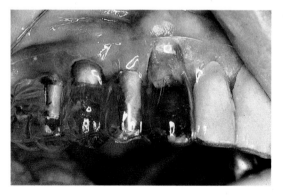

Fig 6-24 Vacuum-formed coping over a cast temporization coping. An access opening has been made in the occlusal surface.

Fig 6-25 The provisional restoration in place. Note screw access channel in the first premolar.

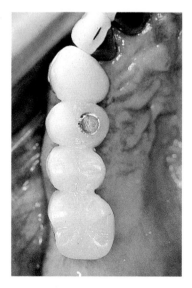

Fig 6-25

Constructing the Prosthesis on the Implant-Abutment Analog

1. Make an impression of the opposing arch, a facebow transfer, and appropriate interocclusal records.
2. Mount casts on a semiadjustable articulator.
3. Select the gold coping. Octagonal gold copings engage the octabutment and are used for single units. Rounded gold copings are used when two or more units are splinted together (Fig 6-26).
4. Place gold copings on the implant abutment analog and attach them with guide screws. Shorten the guide screws as needed for the vertical dimension of occlusion (Fig 6-27). Recut a slot on the occlusal surface of the guide screws.
5. Waxup restoration (Fig 6-28) and invest and cast metal framework (Fig 6-29). For splinted units, a metal try-in is necessary to ensure an accurate passive fit. If the framework rocks or does not fit passively, section the framework and make a soldering index. Resolder and try in the framework once again.

6. The restoration is completed in the laboratory and is ready to be tried in the patient's mouth. The restoration is checked for fit, proximal contacts, contours, and occlusion. Necessary adjustments are made, and the restoration is placed with 4-mm occlusal screws placed hand tight with the occlusal screwdriver (Fig 6-30).
7. Place temporary stopping or cotton over the head of the screw and fill the remainder of the screw access channel with composite resin.
8. For highly divergent implants (greater than 40 degrees) that will be tied together, custom abutments must be fabricated to bring them back into proper alignment (Fig 6-31).

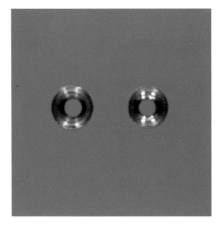

Fig 6-26

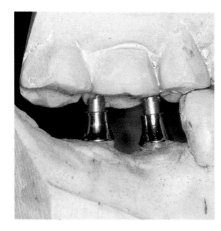

Fig 6-27

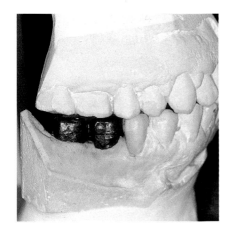

Fig 6-28

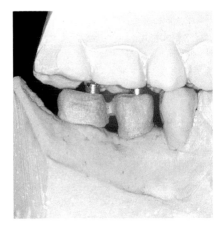

Fig 6-29

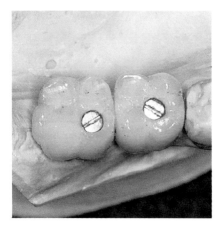

Fig 6-30

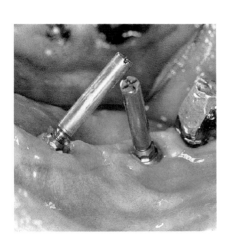

Fig 6-31

Fig 6-26   Gold copings. The octagonal internal design is used for single units to make it nonrotational. The round internal design is used for multiple units that are to be joined.

Fig 6-27   Gold copings in place with the guide screws shortened to occlusal height.

Fig 6-28   The waxup over the gold copings.

Fig 6-29   A metal framework try-in.

Fig 6-30   An occlusal view of the final restorations shows the occlusal screws in place.

Fig 6-31   These two implants had widely divergent pathways. To properly restore these implants, specialized abutment cylinders were fabricated and cast in the laboratory.

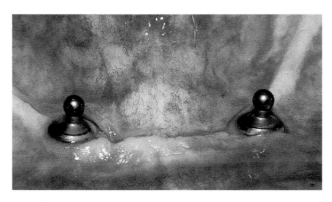

Fig 6-32   Individual retentive anchors have been placed on implants located in the positions previously occupied by the mandibular canines.

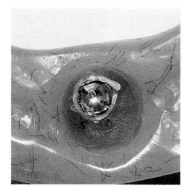

Fig 6-33   The matrix for the retentive anchor Elitor has been placed inside a previously existing denture. (Prosthetics by Dr Norman Dodson.)

Overdentures

Retention for overdentures constructed for ITI implants can be provided by:

- Matrices engaging retentive anchors
- Clips engaging either a round bar or a dolder bar

Retentive anchors may provide less retention than a bar-and-clip overdenture, but they are less complicated to construct and less expensive for the patient.

When two implants are placed in the region of the canines, bar-supported overdentures provide adequate retention and allow rotation of the overdenture around the bar. When implants are placed in the anterior and posterior regions of the mouth, multiple clips can be used, which permits a stable nonrotating and retentive overdenture to be constructed.

Retentive Anchor-Retained Overdenture

If the patient has an acceptable denture that has adequate space for the retentive anchor matrix, and the denture has adequate bulk to resist fracture, the patient's existing denture can be modified.

Direct Approach

1. Remove the closure screw from the implant.
2. Place the retentive anchor hand tight with the retentive anchor driver (Fig 6-32).
3. With the ratchet and retentive anchor driver, tighten the retentive anchor $1/12$ of a turn. This places the retentive anchor at a force of 50 N/cm.
4. Place retentive anchor matrix on the retentive anchor.
5. Relieve the tissue side of the denture in the region of the retentive anchors so that there is 1 mm of space circumferentially around the matrices.

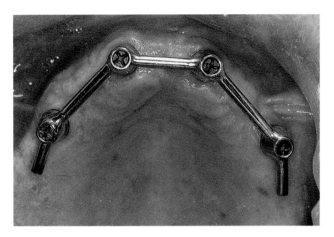

Fig 6-34   The bar in place in the mouth on top of octabutments.

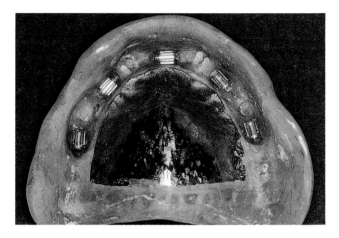

Fig 6-35   The metal substructure has been processed into the denture.

6. Block out undercut areas between the retentive anchor matrix and the retentive anchor abutment. Additionally, the external surface of the matrix should be blocked out except for the mushroom-shaped portion, which is for the retention of the acrylic resin.
7. Add a small amount of autopolymerizing denture base acrylic resin to the tissue side of the denture in the region of the retentive anchors and seat in the patient's mouth.
8. Check stability, fit, and occlusion of the denture.
9. Remove the overdenture from the patient's mouth, adjust the acrylic around the matrices, and adjust the retention of the matrices with the activator or deactivator for matrices as indicated (Fig 6-33).
10. Make periapical radiographs.

Indirect Approach

1. Remove the closure screw from the implant.
2. Place the retentive anchor hand tight with the retentive anchor driver.
3. With the ratchet and retentive anchor driver, tighten the retentive anchor $1/12$ of a turn. This places the retentive anchor at a force of 50 N/cm.
4. Fabricate custom denture impression tray and fit in mouth.
5. Border mold the tray.
6. Make an impression with an elastomeric impression material.
7. Remove impression and place laboratory analog (transfer pin for retentive anchor) into the impression.
8. Pour master cast in die stone.
9. Fabricate records, bases, and occlusion rims, and make jaw relation records and facebow transfer.
10. Mount casts on a semiadjustable articulator.
11. Select prosthetic teeth and set teeth.
12. Wax try-in.
13. Return case to laboratory for fabrication of metal framework and to process and finish the teeth. A metal framework is used when needed for strength.
14. The matrices for retentive anchors may be placed by the laboratory or by the direct approach described above.
15. Deliver denture and check fit and occlusion.
16. Make periapical radiographs.

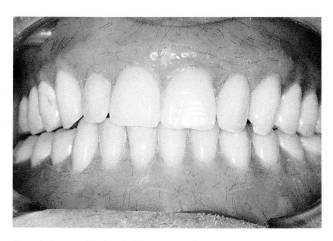

Fig 6-36   The final denture in place. (Courtesy Dr Frank L. Higginbottom.)

Bar-Retained Overdentures

In most cases, the patient's existing denture should not be adapted for bar-retained overdentures because of the space requirements for gold copings and bars and clips, which makes such an overdenture subject to fracture. A metal reinforcement is suggested to add strength to the overdenture.

There are two types of bars available with the ITI system, the round bar and the Dolder bar. The round bar provides more retention than the Dolder bar. The Dolder bar is sometimes preferred because of its ability to act as a stress breaker due to the design of the bar sleeve.

1. Border mold a custom impression tray.
2. Remove the closure screws.
3. Insert octabutments (see page 74).
4. Place transfer copings (see page 74).
5. Make an impression with an elastomeric impression material.
6. Attach implant-abutment analogs to the transfer copings and pour the master cast with die stone.
7. Fabricate the bar splint using either the round bar or Dolder bar and gold copings for overdentures (Fig 6-34).
8. Try in the bar splint and check for good passive fit. If necessary, section the splint, make a soldering index, resolder, and try in the framework once again (Fig 6-35).
9. Make record bases, occlusion rims, a facebow transfer, and a centric relation record, and mount casts on a semiadjustable articulator.
10. Set denture teeth and verify vertical dimension of occlusion, centric relation, and esthetics.
11. Construct a custom-made metal reinforcement for the denture base and process the denture (Fig 6-36).
12. Clips or sleeves may be processed into the overdenture by the laboratory or processed into the overdenture chairside (see page 81 on attaching the matrix to the retentive anchor retained overdenture).

7   IMPLANT MAINTENANCE

A small percentage of implants placed ultimately fail. These appear to fail either from trauma (from the occlusion or an ill-fitting prosthesis) or from an infection, or from a combination of these factors. We do not yet know how often implants fail in the average implant practice, but it is estimated that up to 10% of those implants placed will be lost. A large number of implants will fail early in treatment. Titanium fixtures that fail after prosthetic restoration fail at highly variable rates, but failure appears to be reversible in many cases, which argues for implant maintenance.

At a typical maintenance visit:

1. Update the patient's medical and dental history.
2. Review oral hygiene if needed. The patient should know that:
    • Single-tuft rotating electric toothbrushes work well for cleaning the implant, abutment cylinders, and overlying prostheses.
    • If interproximal brushes are used, the wire should be coated with nylon to avoid scratching the implant.
    • The short-term use of chlorhexidine is often helpful when other methods prove ineffective, as are shortened maintenance intervals.
3. Probe sites (up to six) around each implant using a standardized plastic probe.
    • Record probing depth (from a fixed position, if possible).
    • Record bleeding upon probing or suppuration.
4. Check for signs of trauma from occlusion.
    • Worn prosthesis
    • Loosened screws
    • Broken abutment screws, abutments, or implants
    • Patient complaints of pain in the implant area
5. Check the overlying prosthesis.
6. Remove any tooth-borne material.
    • Use specially designed nonmetallic curettes.
    • Follow with a rubber cup and fine prophylactic paste.
7. Take radiographs, vertical bitewing radiographs, or periapical radiographs once a year (more often in cases with active breakdown).

See the patient as often as necessary to keep the periodontium or periimplant tissues healthy (usually every three months if periodontal disease is present). Totally edentulous patients should be seen at least once per year.

8   TREATMENT OF FAILING IMPLANTS

Prevention

Because implants appear to fail from either trauma or infection (or a combination of these factors), the dental professional can help prevent failure before it occurs or treat these problems before they cause implant failure.

Once tissue integration occurs, failure usually comes slowly to the involved titanium implant, in contrast to hydroxyapatite-coated implants, which can fail very rapidly. As one places more implants, larger numbers (but, hopefully, smaller percentages) will fail. Even with a small percentage of failure, periodic examination and maintenance must occur, because gingival inflammation around implants seems to proceed in a manner similar to that seen around natural teeth.[55,56]

Therapy

The simplest way to treat an implant affected by gingival inflammation is to place the patient on routine maintenance and to reinforce the importance of good personal oral hygiene techniques (see chapter 7). For the patient with progressive tissue loss, treatment is more problematic, and numerous approaches have been suggested. The information that follows is a compilation of early experiences with trying to halt the process of soft and hard tissue loss.

When pocket depths increase and radiographic signs indicate early alveolar deterioration, the clinician should take steps to intervene. Our understanding of these methods is in the early stages of development and answers are not yet available. Trauma should be evaluated and, if present, should be eliminated. This may require anything from occlusal adjustment, to a habit device, to removing the prosthesis. Infection of tissues around implants can often be arrested in the early stages with a combination of mechanical steps (removal of microbes and their products by the patient and the dental therapist) and combined antibiotic and antimicrobial therapy. Mechanical debridement in the early stage takes the form of removal of bacteria and their products with special scalers.

When more advanced tissue loss occurs, debridement is facilitated by the reflection of soft tissue flaps. Treatment of the implant surface can take two forms. (1) When bone has been lost in a horizontal pattern, the chance for success using the principles of guided tissue regeneration (GTR) is reduced. In these cases, the plasma-sprayed surface of the implant can be removed with a high-speed bur and copious irrigation. The remaining surface is polished with fine prophylactic paste and rubber cups. The soft tissues are then apically positioned. (2) When there is vertical loss of bone, the principles of GTR can be used. It is best in these cases to punch a hole in the membrane (with the 3.5-mm or 4.2-mm punch) and drape the membrane around the implant or if possible in other systems to drape the membrane over the implant after the prosthesis has been removed (Figs 8-1 and 8-2). It is also important in these cases to clean the implant surface. Decontamination of the implant is now the subject of great debate, and the best approach has yet to be determined. At present, chlorhexidine is used to clean the implant after any apparent bacteria or their products have been removed from the TPS surface. This is followed by rinsing the surface with sterile saline. Normal GTR procedures are then followed.

Implant failure can take two forms. In the first, the implant becomes mobile and is usually removed gently (Figs 8-3 and 8-4). In the second case, the implant is stable but is deemed a failure by either the dentist or the patient. This failure may be a personal choice by the patient or a professional one by the dentist. Reasons for this type of failure could be uncontrollable infection, continued bone loss, or damage to contiguous structures. The process of removal of ITI implants first involves reducing the diameter of the cervical collar of the implant after the crowns have been removed. This is performed with a high-speed, well-cooled diamond bur before the flaps are reflected. A special explantation trephine is then used to remove the bone circumferentially around the implant. These trephine burs come in two lengths and interval diameters of 4.2 mm and 3.6 mm.[57] After trephining to the desired depth, forceps are used to gently twist the implant, thus fracturing the internal core of bone and allowing removal of the implant.

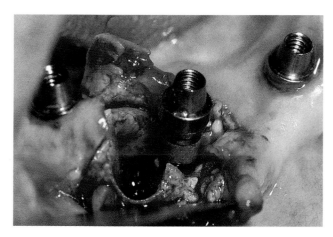

Fig 8-1   A hydroxyapatite-coated implant was placed in direct contact with the root of a canine. Bone breakdown occurred approximately 1.5 years after placement, resulting in the loss of the tooth.

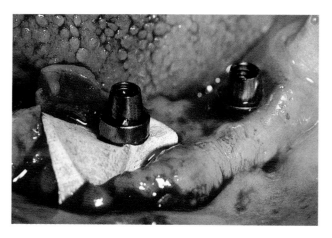

Fig 8-2   After removal of the hydroxyapatite, the implant surface was cleaned with chlorhexidine and an e-PTFE membrane was draped around the fixture. Similar approaches in other cases have provided mixed results, and removal of hydroxyapatite-coated implants that undergo this type of bone loss may be warranted.

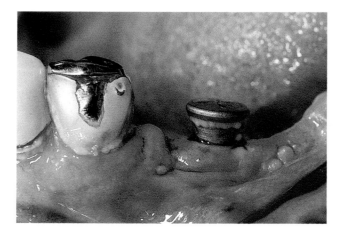

Fig 8-3   This ITI implant had been in place for approximately six months and was apparently well-integrated at the three-month postoperative visit. The patient failed subsequent follow-up visits until she appeared with a chief complaint of tenderness in the area of the implant. The implant, which was mobile, was removed.

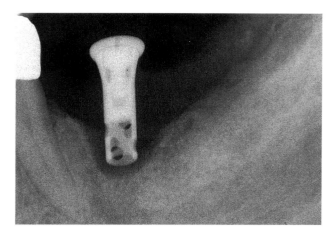

Fig 8-4   Radiograph taken just before the implant seen in Fig 8-3 was removed.

REFERENCES

1. Steinemann S: The properties of titanium. In: Schroeder A, Sutter F, and Krekeler G, eds. *Oral Implantology Basics—ITI Hollow Cylinder System.* Stuttgart: Thieme, 1991, 37–58.

2. Meffert R, Block M, and Kent J: What is osseointegration? *Int J Periodont Rest Dent* 1987;7:9–21.

3. Albrektsson T, Brånemark P-I, Hansson HA, and Lindström J: Osseointegrated titanium implants. *Acta Orthop Scand* 1981;52:155–170.

4. Buser D, Schenk RK, Steinemann S, Fiorellini JP, Fox C, and Stich H: Influence of surface characteristics on bone integration of titanium implants. A histomorphometric study in miniature pigs. *J Biomed Mater Res* 1991;25:889–902.

5. Johnson BW: HA-coated dental implants: Long term consequences. *CDA Journal* 1992;20(6):33.

6. Kirsch A and Donath K: Tierexperimentelle untersuchungen zur bedeutung der micromorphologie von titanimplantatobetichen. *Fortschr Zahnarztl Implantol* 1984;1:35–40.

7. Wilke HJ, Claes L, and Steinemann S: The influence of various titanium surfaces on the interface shear strength between implants and bone. *Adv Biomat* 1990;9:309–314.

8. Buser D, Weber HP, Donath K, Fiorellini JP, Paquette DW, and Williams RC: Soft tissue reactions to nonsubmerged unloaded titanium implants in beagle dogs. *J Periodontol* 1992;63: 226–236.

9. Gotfredsen K, Hjorting-Hansen E, and Budtz-Jorgensen E: Clinical and radiographic evaluation of submerged implants in monkeys. *Int J Prosthodont* 1990;3(5):463–469.

10. Weber HP, Buser D, Donath K et al: Histomorphometry of tissues around submerged and nonsubmerged implants. *J Dent Res* 1992;71:1198.

11. Jaffin RA and Berman CL: The excessive loss of Brånemark fixtures in Type IV bone: A 5-year analysis. *J Periodontol* 1991;62:2–4.

12. Buser D, Weber HP, Bragger U, and Balsiger C: Tissue integration of one-stage ITI implants: 3-year results of a longitudinal study with hollow-cylinder and hollow-screw implants. *Int J Oral Maxillofac Implants* 1991;6(4):405–412.

13. Buser D, Weber HP, and Lang NP: Tissue integration of non-submerged implants: 1-year results of a prospective study with 100 ITI hollow-cylinder and hollow-screw implants. *Clin Oral Impl Res* 1990;1:33–40.

14. Babbush CA, Kent JN, and Misiek DJ: Titanium plasma-sprayed (TPS) screw implants for the reconstruction of the edentulous mandible. *J Oral Maxillofac Surg* 1986;44: 274–282.

15. Sutter F, Schroeder A, and Buser DA: The new concept of ITI hollow-cylinder and hollow-screw implants: Part 1. Engineering and design. *Int J Oral Maxillofac Implants* 1988;3(3): 161–172.

16. Bodine RI and Yanase RT: Thirty-year report on 28 implant dentures inserted between 1952 and 1959. In: *Proceedings of the International Symposium on Preprosthetic Surgery.* Palm Springs, California: 1985.

17. Smithloff M and Fritz ME: The use of blade implants in a selected population of partially edentulous adults. A ten-year report. *J Periodontol* 1982;53:413.

18. Brånemark P-I, Breine U, Adell R, Hansson BO, Lindström J, and Olsson A: Osseointegrated implants in the treatment of the edentulous jaw. Experience from a 10-year period. *Scand J Plast Reconstr Surg* 1977;11(Suppl 16):1–132.

19. Schroeder A, Pohler O, and Sutter F: Gewebsreaktion auf ein Titan-Hohlzylinder implantat mit Titan-Spritzschichtoberflache. *Schweiz Mschr Zahnheilk* 1976;86(7):713–727.

20. Buser D: Current Issues Forum. *Int J Oral Maxillofac Implants* 1992;7:419.

21. Babbush CA, Kent JN, and Salon JM: A solution for the problematic atrophic mandible: The titanium plasma spray (TPS) screw implant system. *Gerodontics* 1986;2:16–23.

22. Adell R, Lekholm U, Rockler B, and Brånemark P-I: A 15-year study of osseointegrated implants in the treatment of the edentulous jaw. *Int J Oral Surg* 1981;10(6):387–416.

23. Mombelli A, Van Oosten MA, Schurch E Jr, and Lang NP: The microbiota associated with successful or failing osseointegrated titanium implants. *Oral Microbiol Immunol* 1987; 2(4):145–151.

24. Kalykakis GK, Yildirim M, Spiekermann H, Nisengard RJ, and Zafiropoulos GGK: Clinical and microbiological status of stable Brånemark implants. In: *Proceedings of the American Academy of Periodontology Annual Meeting.* Orlando, FL: American Academy of Periodontology; 1992.

25. Malmstrom HS, Fritz ME, Timmis DP, and Van Dyke TE: Osseo-integrated implant treatment of a patient with rapidly progressive periodontitis—A case report. *J Periodontol* 1990;61(5):300–304.

26. Higuchi KW and Slack JM: The use of titanium fixtures for intraoral anchorage to facilitate orthodontic tooth movement. *Int J Oral Maxillofac Implants* 1991;6:344.

27. ten Bruggenkate CM, Sutter F, Oosterbeek HS, and Schroeder A: Indications for angled implants. *J Prosthetic Dent* 1992;67(1):85–93.

28. Lang NP and Wilson TG Jr: Choice of implant system and clinical management. In: Wilson TG Jr, Kornman KS, and Newman MG, eds. *Advances in Periodontics.* Chicago: Quintessence; 1992; 370.

29. Brånemark PI: Introduction to osseointegration. In: Brånemark PI, Zarb GA, and Albrektsson T, eds. *Tissue-Integrated Prostheses.* Chicago: Quintessence; 1985; 11.

30. Schroeder A, van der Zypen E, Stich H, and Sutter F: The reactions of bone, connective tissue, and epithelium to endosteal implants with titanium-sprayed surfaces. *J Maxillofac Surg* 1981;9(1):15–25.

31. Eriksson AR and Albrektsson T: Temperature threshold levels for heat-induced bone tissue injury. A vital microscopic study in the rabbit. *J Prosthet Dent* 1983;50:101–107.

32. Sutter F, Krekeler G, Schwammberger AF, and Sutter FJ: Atraumatic surgical technique and implant bed preparation. *Quintessence Int* 1992;23:811–816.

33. Brunski JB, Moccia AF, Pollack SR, Korostoff E, and Trachingbery DI: The influence of functional use of endosseous dental implants on the tissue-implant interface. I. Histological aspects. *J Dent Res* 1979;58:1953–1969.

34. Kasemo B and Lausmaa J: Metal selection and surface characteristics. In: Brånemark PI, Zarb GA, and Albrektsson T, eds. *Tissue-Integrated Prostheses.* Chicago: Quintessence; 1985; 111.

35. Carlsson GE, Bergman B, and Hedegard B: Changes in contour of the maxillary alveolar process under immediate dentures. A longitudinal clinical and x-ray cephalometric study covering 5 years. *Acta Odontol Scand* 1967;25:1.

36. Carlsson GE and Persson G: Morphologic changes of the mandible after extraction and wearing of dentures. *Odont Revy* 1967;18:27.

37. Bergman B and Carlsson GE: Clinical long-term study of complete denture wearers. *J Prosthetic Dent* 1985;53:56–61.

38. Atwood DA: Reduction of residual ridges: A major oral disease entity. *J Prosthet Dent* 1971;26:266.

39. Tallgren A: Continuing reduction of residual alveolar ridges in complete denture wearers: Mixed longitudinal study covering 25 years. *J Prosthet Dent* 1972;27:120.

40. Nicol BR, Somes GW, Ellinger CW, Unger JW, and Fuhrman J: Patient response to variations in denture technique. Part II: Five-year cephalometric evaluation. *J Prosthet Dent* 1979;41:368.

41. Clarke MA and Bueltmann KW: Anatomical considerations in periodontal surgery. *J Periodontol* 1971;42:610–625.

42. Westmoreland FF and Blanton PL: An analysis of the variations in positions of the greater palatine foramen in the adult human skull. *Anat Rec* 1982;204:383–388.

43. Wilson C: *Lingual Nerve: Anatomic Relationship to the Mandibular Alveolar Crest and Lingual Cortical Plate.* Thesis, Baylor College of Dentistry, Dallas, Texas, 1989.

44. Rajchel J, Ellis E, and Fonseca RJ: The anatomical location of the mandibular canal: Its relationship to the sagittal ramus osteotomy. *Int J Adult Orthod Orthognath Surg* 1986;1:37–47.

45. Heasman PA: Variation in the position of the inferior dental canal and its significance to restorative dentistry. *J Dent* 1988;16:36–39.

46. Matheson BR: *Localization of the Mental Foramen Utilizing an Intraoral Landmark.* Thesis, Baylor College of Dentistry, Dallas, Texas, 1985.

47. Dmytryk JJ, Fox SC, and Moriarty JD: The effects of scaling titanium implant surfaces with metal and plastic instruments on cell attachment. *J Periodontol* 1990;61:491–496.

48. Nyman S, Lindhe J, Karring T, and Rylander H: New attachment following surgical treatment of human periodontal disease. *J Clin Periodontol* 1982;4(4):290–296.

49. Dahlin C, Sennerby L, Lekholm U, Linde A, and Nyman S: Generation of new bone around titanium implants using a membrane technique: An experimental study in rabbits. *Int J Oral Maxillofac Implants* 1989;4(1):19–25.

50. Novaes AB and Novaes AB: IMZ implants placed into extraction sockets in association with membrane therapy (Gengiflex) and porous hydroxyapatite. A case report. *Int J Oral Maxillofac Implants* 1992;7:536–540.

51. Balshi TJ, Hernandez RE, Cutler RH, and Hertzog CF: Treatment of osseous defects using Vycril mesh (Polyglactin 910) and the Brånemark implant. *Int J Oral Maxillofac Implants* 1991;6:87–91.

52. Wilson TG and Weber HP: Classification and therapy for areas of deficient bony housing prior to dental implant placement. *Int J Periodontol Rest Dent* 1993;13:(5).

53. Cochran DL and Douglas H: Augmentation of osseous tissue around nonsubmerged endosseous dental implants. *Int J Periodontal Rest Dent*; In Press.

54. Buser D, Brägger U, Lang NP, and Nyman S: Regeneration and enlargement of jaw bone using guided tissue regeneration. *Clin Oral Implant Res* 1990;1:22–32.

55. Lindhe J, Marinello C, Ericsson I, and Liljenberg B: Soft tissue reaction to de novo plaque formation on implants and teeth. An experimental study in the dog. *Clin Oral Implant Res* 1992;3:1–8.

56. Lindhe J, Berglundh T, Ericsson I, Liljenberg B, and Marinello C: Experimental breakdown of peri-implant and periodontal tissues. A study in the beagle dog. *Clin Oral Implant Res* 1992;3:9–16.

57. ten Bruggenkate CM, Sutter F, Schroder A, and Oosterbook HS: Explantation procedure in the F-Typor and bone fit ITI implant system. In: ten Bruggenkate CM, eds. *Clinical and Radiological Aspects of Oral Implants, With Special Emphasis on the ITI Hollow Cylinder Implant.* 'S-Gravenhage: Pasmans Offsetdrukkerij; 1990; 153–159.

CASE PRESENTATIONS

This chapter presents before-and-after images that can be used effectively in patient consultations. These case presentations demonstrate how implant restorations look, as well as the many situations in which implant-borne prostheses may be used.

Acknowledgments

Case 1. Restorative dentistry courtesy Dr John Michael Kidwell, laboratory work by Singler Dental Ceramics, Dallas, Texas.

Case 2. Restorative dentistry courtesy Dr Frank L. Higginbottom, laboratory work by Singler Dental Ceramics.

Case 3. Restorative dentistry courtesy Dr Douglas Martin, metal framework by RK Dental Laboratory, Tuscola, Texas, ceramics by Trinity Dental Studios, Flower Mound, Texas.

Case 4. Restorative dentistry courtesy Dr Frank L. Higginbottom, laboratory work by Singler Dental Ceramics.

Case 5. Restorative dentistry courtesy Dr Frank L. Higginbottom, laboratory work by Singler Dental Ceramics.

Case 6. Restorative dentistry courtesy Dr John Michael Kidwell, laboratory work by Singler Dental Ceramics.

Case 7. Restorative dentistry courtesy Dr R. Norman Dodson, laboratory work by Function Esthetics, Lewisville, Texas.

Case 8. Restorative dentistry Dr R. Norman Dodson, laboratory work by Function Esthetics.

Case 1

A lower canine is replaced with an implant. The crown is not attached to the adjacent teeth.

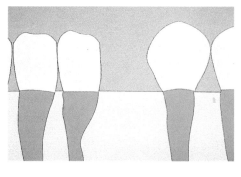
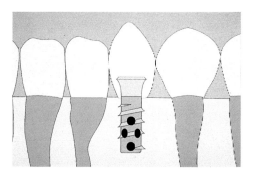
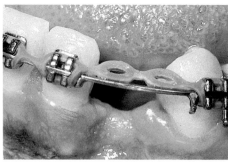
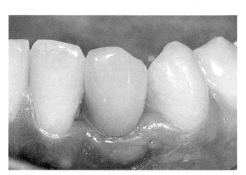

Case 2

A lower molar is replaced with an implant. The crown is not attached to the adjacent teeth.

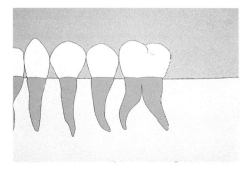
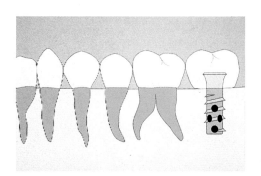
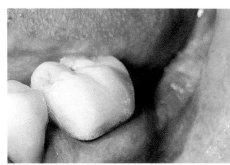
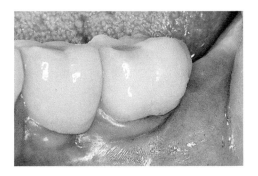

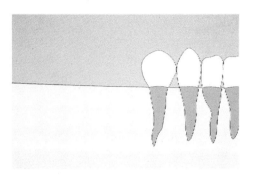

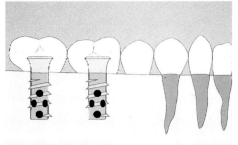

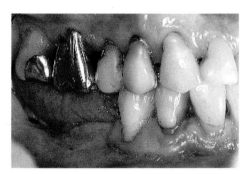

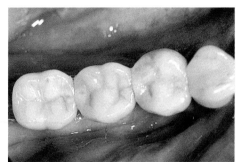

Case 3

Teeth are replaced on the lower right side with crowns on two implants. The crowns are attached only to the implants, and a pontic (dummy tooth) has been set in the space in front of the implants.

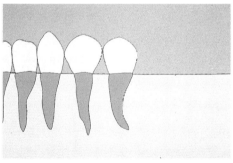

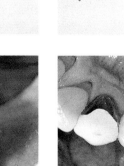

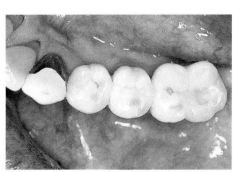

Case 4

The second tooth from the right was removed because of severe tooth decay (top right). The crowns are attached to both the implant and to the adjacent natural teeth.

Case 5

Two of the patient's teeth broke off. Two implants were placed. For additional strength, the crowns are attached to both the implants and to the adjacent natural teeth.

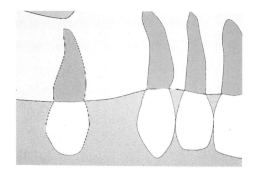
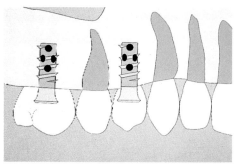
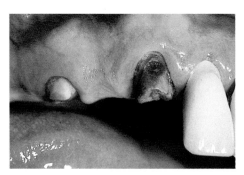
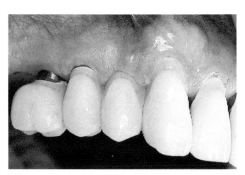

Case 6

This patient's teeth were prepared to hold a temporary bridge, which the patient wore while his implants healed. The final crowns are attached to both the implants and the natural teeth.

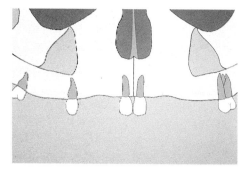
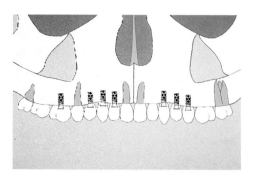
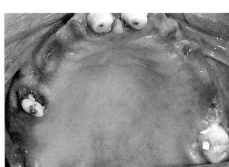
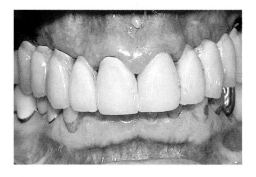

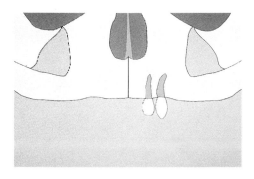
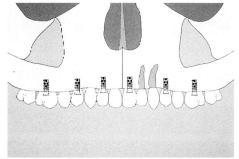

Case 7

These crowns are attached to both the implants and to the two natural teeth. The lips cover the gums and adjacent parts of the teeth during normal facial expressions.

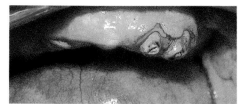
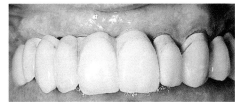

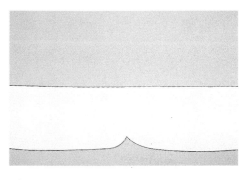
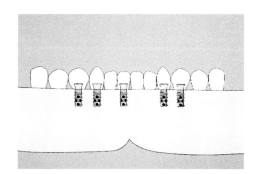

Case 8

Implants were placed in this patient's lower jaw, which was entirely without teeth. The spaces below the restoration, which allow the patient to clean the area, do not show during normal facial expressions.

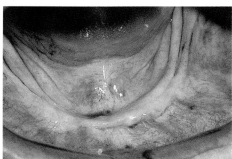
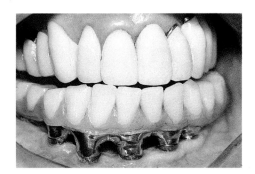